MORE PRAISE FOR
JOHNS HOPKINS PATIENTS'
GUIDE TO OVARIAN CANCER

"Drs. Bristow and Salani have done an outstanding job of providing ovarian cancer patients and their families with exactly what they need: a well-written and thoughtful approach to dealing with all aspects of ovarian cancer *from the patient's perspective*. In this clear and easily understandable document, a patient can find the comprehensive, up-to-date information she needs to approach this disease in a confident and knowledgeable fashion. This resource goes a long way in providing guidance for ovarian cancer patients and their families in managing this disease."

> Laurel W. Rice, MD
> Professor and Chair
> The University of Wisconsin School of Medicine and Public Health
> Madison, Wisconsin

"Should I have a family member with the diagnosis of ovarian cancer, I would strongly recommend she read this guide. Unquestionably, she would benefit from the knowledge and guidance provided in this concise and well-written patient guide. The information is contemporary and comprehensive, offering the ovarian cancer patient a blueprint of how to be in control of the management of her health care. Bravo to Drs. Bristow and Salani for providing this greatly needed resource."

> Larry J. Copeland, MD
> The William Greenville Pace III and Joann Norris Collins-Pace
> Chair for Cancer Research
> Professor and Chair
> Department of Obstetrics and Gynecology
> The James Cancer Hospital and Solove Research Insititute
> Ohio State University
> Columbus, Ohio

"A diagnosis of cancer can turn one's world upside down. This comprehensive, practical, and easy-to-read *Patient's Guide to Ovarian Cancer* can help bring a sense of control to an often overwhelming situation for both patients and their families. It will be a great asset, providing clarity in often cloudy circumstances."

Lois M. Ramondetta, MD
Associate Professor
Department of Gynecologic Oncology
The University of Texas MD Anderson Cancer Center
Houston, Texas
Co-author of *The Light Within: The Extraordinary Friendship of a Doctor and Patient Brought Together by Cancer*, William Morrow Publisher (www.thelightwithinbook.com)

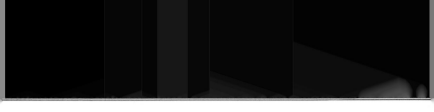

Patients' Guide to
Ovarian Cancer

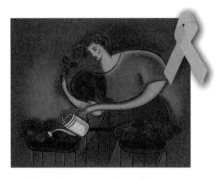

Ritu Salani, MD, MBA

Assistant Professor, Division of Gynecologic Oncology, Department of Obstetrics & Gynecology
The James Cancer Hospital and Solove Research Institute
The Ohio State University College of Medicine

Robert E. Bristow, MD, MBA

Director, Kelly Gynecologic Oncology Service
Professor, Department of Gynecology and Obstetrics, Johns Hopkins School of Medicine

SERIES EDITORS
Lillie D. Shockney, RN, BS, MAS

University Distinguished Service Assistant Professor of Breast Cancer; Administrative Director of Breast
Cancer; Assistant Professor, Department of Surgery; Assistant Professor, Department of Obstetrics and
Gynecology, Johns Hopkins School of Medicine; Assistant Professor, Johns Hopkins School of Nursing

Gary R. Shapiro, MD

Chairman, Department of Oncology
Johns Hopkins Bayview Medical Center
Director, Johns Hopkins Geriatric Oncology Program
The Sidney Kimmel Comprehensive Cancer Center at Johns Hopkins

JONES AND BARTLETT PUBLISHERS
Sudbury, Massachusetts
BOSTON   TORONTO   LONDON   SINGAPORE

World Headquarters

Jones and Bartlett Publishers
40 Tall Pine Drive
Sudbury, MA 01776
978-443-5000
info@jbpub.com
www.jbpub.com

Jones and Bartlett Publishers
Canada
6339 Ormindale Way
Mississauga, Ontario L5V 1J2
Canada

Jones and Bartlett Publishers
International
Barb House, Barb Mews
London W6 7PA
United Kingdom

Jones and Bartlett's books and products are available through most bookstores and online booksellers. To contact Jones and Bartlett Publishers directly, call 800-832-0034, fax 978-443-8000, or visit our website, www.jbpub.com.

Substantial discounts on bulk quantities of Jones and Bartlett's publications are available to corporations, professional associations, and other qualified organizations. For details and specific discount information, contact the special sales department at Jones and Bartlett via the above contact information or send an email to specialsales@jbpub.com.

The authors, editor, and publisher have made every effort to provide accurate information. However, they are not responsible for errors, omissions, or for any outcomes related to the use of the contents of this book and take no responsibility for the use of the products and procedures described. Treatments and side effects described in this book may not be applicable to all people; likewise, some people may require a dose or experience a side effect that is not described herein. Drugs and medical devices are discussed that may have limited availability controlled by the Food and Drug Administration (FDA) for use only in a research study or clinical trial. Research, clinical practice, and government regulations often change the accepted standard in this field. When consideration is being given to use of any drug in the clinical setting, the healthcare provider or reader is responsible for determining FDA status of the drug, reading the package insert, and reviewing prescribing information for the most up-to-date recommendations on dose, precautions, and contraindications, and determining the appropriate usage for the product. This is especially important in the case of drugs that are new or seldom used.

Production Credits
Publisher: Christopher Davis
Editorial Assistant: Sara Cameron
Production Director: Amy Rose
Production Assistant: Tina Chen
Senior Marketing Manager: Barb Bartoszek
V.P., Manufacturing and Inventory Control: Therese Connell
Cover Design: Kristin E. Parker
Cover Image: © Image Club Graphics
Composition: Publishers' Design and Production Services, Inc.
Printing and Binding: Malloy, Inc.
Cover Printing: Malloy, Inc.

Library of Congress Cataloging-in-Publication Data
Salani, Ritu.
    Johns Hopkins patients' guide to ovarian cancer / Ritu Salani, Robert E. Bristow.
      p. cm.
    Includes index.
    ISBN 978-0-7637-7437-0
1. Ovaries—Cancer—Popular works.   I. Johns Hopkins Medicine. II. Title. III. Title: Patients' guide to ovarian cancer.
    RC280.O8B75 2009
    616.99'465—dc22

                                                                                    2009024207

6048

Printed in the United States of America
13 12 11 10 09   10 9 8 7 6 5 4 3 2 1

Contents

Introduction

How to Use This Book to Your Benefit

You will receive a great deal of information from your healthcare team. You will also probably seek some information out on the Internet or in the bookstores. No doubt friends and family members, meaning well, will attempt to give you advice on what to do and when to do it, and try to steer you in certain directions. Relax. Yes, you have heard words you wish you had never heard said about you, that you have ovarian cancer. Despite that shocking phrase, you have time to make good decisions and to empower yourself with accurate information so that you can participate in the decision making about your care and treatment.

This book is designed to be a "how-to" guide in taking you through the maze of treatment options and sometimes complicated schedules, and will help you put together a plan of action so that you become an ovarian cancer survivor.

You will note that the book is broken down into chapters. Chapter 11 is an index of credible resources listed for your further review and education. By empowering yourself with accurate and understandable information, you are in a much better position to be able to make treatment decisions with your doctors rather than have your doctors make them for you without your understanding how, when, or why.

There is a natural sense of urgency to proceed with surgery and possibly chemotherapy as soon as possible when you have a possible or definite diagnosis of ovarian cancer. However, the intial decision you make about where to receive treatment and from which multidisciplinary team can be crucial to determining the overall treatment outcome. This book will give you the information and tools you need to make informed decisions in a timely manner to ensure that you give yourself the best chance for a good outcome and beating ovarian cancer.

Let's begin now with understanding what has happened and what the steps are to get you well again.

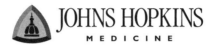
JOHNS HOPKINS
MEDICINE

FIRST STEPS—
I'VE BEEN DIAGNOSED
WITH OVARIAN CANCER

O varian cancer is a relatively uncommon disease. Still, in the United States, it occurs in approximately 1 in 55 women. This is an estimated 23,000 women per year and it is the cause of death in over 16,000 women per year.

The cancer starts in the ovaries, which are the hormone secreting organs of the reproductive system. These hormones, which include estrogen, progesterone, and androgens, are responsible for sexual development, inducing the menstrual cycle, and release of the egg (oocyte) that can be fertilized to result in pregnancy.

Ovarian cancer can develop from different components of the ovary. The most common type is epithelial ovarian cancer, which arises from the lining of the ovarian surface. Within this group are subcategories that are determined by the pathologist after microscopic examination. These subcategories include serous (most common), mucinous, endometrioid, and clear cell. Less common types of ovarian cancer include germ cell tumors and sex-cord stromal tumors. Germ cell tumors originate from the cells responsible for producing the oocyte. Sex-cord stromal tumors arise from the surrounding connective tissue of the ovary, also known as the stroma.

There is also a group of epithelial tumors that fall in between benign (noncancerous) tumors and cancer. These tumors have several different names and may be referred to as borderline ovarian tumors, tumors of low malignant potential, or atypical proliferative ovarian tumors. Although these types of tumors have some properties of malignancy, such as the ability to recur, they are not considered invasive cancer. If you would like more information on any of the tumor types described above, we recommend Web sites such as that of the National Cancer Institute (**http://www .cancer.gov**) and the National Comprehensive Cancer Network (**http://www.nccn.org**).

Once medical care is sought for a suspected or confirmed diagnosis of ovarian cancer, a full history and physical should be obtained by the provider. Although a pelvic examination is a crucial part of the evaluation, it may not be sensitive enough to detect ovarian cancer. Further investigation may be carried out with a pelvic ultrasound, computerized axial tomography (CAT scan), or magnetic resonance imaging (MRI). However, these techniques do not provide a definitive diagnosis and surgical evaluation may be necessary to confirm the presence of the disease. This may range from a diagnostic laparoscopy to an open abdominal exploration.

RISK FACTORS

There are some characteristics that may place a woman at a higher risk for developing ovarian cancer than the average woman. These risks can be divided into two major categories. The first of which is incessant ovulation. This means that a woman releases an egg from her ovaries each month, without interruption. The theory behind this concept is that the ovary has to repair itself every time the egg is released. The more often this repair occurs, the more likely the chance of a genetic mutation occurring. This genetic mutation then results in the formation of an ovarian cancer. Events that fall into this category include starting menses at an early age (menarche), undergoing menopause at a later age, and few or no pregnancies. There are also factors that can reduce your risk of ovarian cancer by preventing incessant ovulation. This includes breast feeding and use of birth control pills, which have been shown to reduce the risk of ovarian cancer by 50% if taken for five years.

The other category includes genetic predisposition for ovarian cancer and a strong family history. Genetic predisposition is the inheritance of a mutation in a gene that results in abnormal DNA and, thus, abnormal cellular function. There are two main types of genetic mutations that result in cancer. The first is the loss of a gene that prevents cancer cells from overgrowing; these genes are referred to as tumor suppressor genes. Examples of this type of gene include BRCA1 and BRCA2. The other type of mutation that

3

may results in a cancer is an oncogene, or a gene that stimulates cell growth. Although genetics play an important role in ovarian cancer, this comprises approximately 10% of all cases. Other risk factors include increasing age and demographic factors such as European/Northern American descent and high socioeconomic status.

SYMPTOMS AND DIAGNOSIS

The majority of patients with ovarian cancer present in advanced stages. The reasons are multifold. First, as of yet there is no screening test that allows for detection in early phases of the disease, such as mammography for breast cancers or colonoscopy for colon cancers. Secondly, there are no distinctive symptoms that cause one to suspect ovarian cancer. Symptoms associated with ovarian cancer are often vague and may not cause one to seek medical care. These symptoms include the following: increasing abdominal size, abdominal bloating, fatigue, abdominal pain, indigestion, constipation, and urinary symptoms. Up to one-third of women reported having these symptoms for more than six months prior to the diagnosis. Therefore, it is important to seek medical care if you experience these symptoms or others persist.

SELECTING AN ONCOLOGIST AND MEDICAL CENTER

Once a diagnosis of ovarian cancer is suspected or made, it is critical to find the right team. The first step is to seek the opinion of a gynecologic oncologist. Multiple studies have shown that a woman is more likely to undergo the proper staging procedures if the surgery is performed by a gynecologic oncologist rather than a general gynecologist or a general surgeon. Locating a gynecologic oncologist may be done by finding a comprehensive cancer center or looking on the

Internet at sites such as the National Comprehensive Cancer Network (**http://www.nccn.org/index.asp**), the National Cancer Institute (NCI: **http://cancercenters.cancer.gov/**), the Women's Cancer Network (WCN; **http://www.wcn.org/about/gcf.html**), Cancer*Care* (**http://www.cancercare.org**), and Emory Healthcare (**http://www.emoryhealthcare.org**). A list of trusted resources can be found in Chapter 11.

It is important to understand the treatment philosophy of the gynecologic oncologist. You are encouraged to ask several questions of your physician. Is he/she board eligible or certified in the field of gynecologic oncology? How many ovarian cancer cases does he/she perform each year? What is his/her optimal cytoreduction rate (discussed in more detail on page 21)? Does he/she administer chemotherapy? These are just several of the questions you should ask prior to undergoing treatment. If you are not comfortable with the answers you have received or would like more information, a second opinion may be helpful.

LEARNING ABOUT YOUR DISEASE BEFORE THE FIRST VISIT

Being diagnosed with cancer is a life-changing event. There are several things you should know about ovarian cancer prior to entering the office.

Being treated by a gynecologic oncologist will provide you the best chances for survival. Although a majority of ovarian cancers are diagnosed at more advanced stages, approximately 80% of women will have a response to the chemotherapy. There are excellent medications available to help prevent many of the side effects from chemotherapy. Women can continue their normal daily activities during the treatment process.

GATHERING RECORDS, BIOPSY, LABS, RADIOLOGY REPORTS, OTHER TESTS

It is important that you obtain any studies that provide insight into the status of the disease. This includes the actual images of any radiographic imaging, such as an ultrasound, computed axial tomography (CAT) scan, or magnetic resonance imaging (MRI). Obtain the slides of any specimens such as pathology, if biopsies were performed, or cytology, if fluid collections were sampled; these include ascites (fluid in the abdomen) or pleural effusion (fluid around the lungs) if not done at the treating institution. This allows the specialists—both the gynecologic oncologist and pathologist—to review the accuracy of the diagnosis.

It is recommended that you keep a copy of your medical records throughout your care. Any time you see a new physician regarding your ovarian cancer care, you should bring your records with you for their review.

CANCER STAGING

Staging of cancer is performed in order to determine the extent and spread of the disease. The stage may determine the type of treatment administered as well as the overall prognosis from the disease. Once ovarian cancer is diagnosed or suspected, the next step usually involves undergoing a staging procedure. Ovarian cancer is surgically staged, meaning one must undergo a surgical operation in order to determine the extent and spread of the disease. Typically, the diagnosis and the staging procedure are done at the same time. A majority of women are found to have advanced disease at the time of diagnosis.

OVARIAN CANCER STAGING IS BASED ON THE
INTERNATIONAL FEDERATION OF GYNECOLOGY
AND OBSTETRICS (FIGO)

Stage I: The cancer spread is limited to one or both ovaries

IA: Disease is confined to one ovary

IB: Disease is confined to both ovaries

IC: Stage IA or IB with cancer cells on the ovarian surface, cancer cells in the peritoneal washings or ascites, or rupture of the ovarian tumor

Stage II: The cancer is confined to the pelvis

IIA: Disease has spread to the fallopian tubes and/or uterus

IIB: Disease involves other pelvic organs including the bladder, pelvic colon, or peritoneum

IIC: Stage IIA or IIB with cancer cells on the ovarian surface, pelvic washings or ascites, or rupture of the ovarian tumor

Stage III: The cancer has spread to the abdomen

IIIA: Microscopic disease in the abdominal cavity

IIIB: Abdominal disease that is 2 cm or less in diameter

IIIC: Abdominal disease that is greater than 2 cm or spread to the retroperitoneal lymph nodes (pelvic, para-aortic, or inguinal)

Stage IV: Spread of disease outside of the abdomen such as a positive pleural effusion (cancer cells in the fluid surrounding the lung) or involvement of the liver parenchyma (tumor in the internal portion of the liver)

OK, now that you have been told that you may have ovarian cancer or have already been given your diagnosis, take a deep breath. There is going to be a lot of information for you to retain and much of it will be very confusing. By the end of the process, you will be quite comfortable with the language of the disease as well as the treatment philosophies. Until that point, make every effort to ask questions and understand what's happening to your body. Try not to get ahead of yourself—many questions you may have will be answered as the process continues.

In addition to the type of tumor (such as epithelial, germ cell, or sex-cord stromal tumors), further microscopic examination can reveal the degree of differentiation of the tumor. This essentially means how closely the cancer cells resemble the normal cells. The term well-differentiated means that the cancer cells resemble the normal cells of the ovary. Cancer cells that have lost any resemblance to normal cells are referred to as poorly-differentiated, these cells tend to be more aggressive then cells from well-differentiated tumors. Occasionally the differentiation is referred to as the grade of the tumor. Grades can be described as the following:

- Grade 1 is well-differentiated; these cells tend to be slow growing.

- Grade 2 is moderately-differentiated; these cells act somewhere in between well and poorly-differentiated tumors.

- Grade 3 is poorly-differentiated; these cells are rapidly growing.

Having a grade 3 tumor is common. It is a relative term and does not indicate that your tumor is uncontrollable. Grade and stage describe two different components of the tumor. Grade is related to the rate of cell growth or "aggressiveness" of the tumor. Stage describes the extent or spread of the disease. Although both grade and stage may provide information about survival rates, it is important to remember that each individual, such as yourself, is not controlled by these statistics.

GENETICS OF OVARIAN CANCER

Approximately 10% of women who develop ovarian cancers have a genetic predisposition. Although this is a relatively small percentage, it is still important to recognize the risks as many of these cases may be preventable. Women with multiple family members with ovarian or breast cancer, particularly first degree relatives (mother, sisters, daughters) may have a genetic risk. Another indication of a possible genetic cause is the development of ovarian cancer at an early age, particularly premenopausally.

If you have a strong family history, or have had family members or you yourself were diagnosed at a young age, you should consider seeking genetic counseling. These counselors will review your family history and provide a risk assessment. They may also offer you genetic testing if potentially beneficial. This consists of a blood test that is used to analyze specific genes in your DNA to determine the presence or absence of two genes known as BRCA1 and BRCA2. These genes are associated with both breast and ovarian cancer. The risk of ovarian cancer may be as high as 40% in women with these mutations. Although more common in women of Jewish descent (particularly eastern European), the mutation can be found in anyone.

Another genetic syndrome associated with ovarian cancer is hereditary nonpolyposis colorectal cancer (HNPCC). This syndrome is associated with colorectal cancer and endometrial cancer as well as several other types of cancers. It can be tested for by an analysis of cancerous tissue that has been removed. The tests may help provide an understanding of why you developed ovarian cancer, determine what your risk is for other types of cancer, and provide a risk assessment for family members. It is important to understand the results, both negative and positive. The test results may imply that you have a high risk of developing breast cancer. Then you would have to consider how aggressively you would want to approach this type of situation; this may range from taking anti-estrogen therapy to prophylactic surgery. Additionally, you may want to talk to family members about how your test results may affect them. Even if you have a strong family history, you may have a negative test result. This doesn't mean that there isn't a genetic link, but rather that the gene may not have been identified yet. Meeting with a genetic counselor and reviewing your history, regardless of the test result, may give you a better understanding of your cancer.

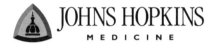

CHAPTER 2

MY TEAM—MEETING YOUR TREATMENT TEAM

TEAM MEMBERS

Your oncology team begins with your diagnosis and consists of many members from different areas. Each person plays a key role that is instrumental in helping you deal with the many facets of ovarian cancer care. Below is a description of the major team members:

Gynecologic oncologist. This is usually the first doctor that you will see. The gynecologic oncologist is a subspecialist who spends an additional 3 to 4 years of training in dealing with cancer arising from the ovary, uterus, cervix, vagina, and vulva after finishing his or her residency in obstetrics and gynecology. They are trained in removing lymph nodes, performing radical surgery, and administering chemotherapy.

Medical oncologist. You will see this specialist if you require any chemotherapy treatment unless your gynecologic oncologist is trained to do this. A medical oncologist is a doctor who specializes in diagnosing and treating cancer using chemotherapy, hormonal therapy, and biological therapy. A medical oncologist often is the main healthcare provider for someone who has cancer. A medical oncologist also gives supportive care and may coordinate treatment given by other specialists. Some medical oncologists specialize in gynecologic cancer. The consultation with this doctor is usually 1 to 2 weeks after your surgery is completed and when the final pathology results are available. Medical oncologists work in conjunction with gynecologic oncologists in laying out your treatment plan.

Nurses. Several are involved in your care from the beginning. Initially, you will work with surgical nurses and floor nurses throughout your hospital stay. Once the diagnosis and stage are confirmed, you will meet with the chemotherapy nurses. They help to coordinate your care during this phase, including education on the medications, the administration of the drugs, and scheduling of laboratory/radiology tests.

Nutritionist. This degreed professional may be consulted to help you obtain your nutritional needs during your postoperative healing period as well as during your chemotherapy course.

Pathologist. This is a "behind the scenes" physician specialist who reviews your tissue specimens by looking under the microscope. He or she decides what type of ovarian cancer you have, and will grade the tumor as well as define the extent/spread of the tumor.

Social worker. This degreed and licensed professional helps coordinate any personal needs you may have, from assisting with financial issues, to arranging for home health care (if necessary), to linking you with support networks and other services.

Surgical intensivist. After your surgery you may require a short stay in the intensive care unit. The surgical intensivist is the physician who will monitor your care along with the gynecologic oncologist.

MAKING YOUR INITIAL APPOINTMENT

For your first appointment regarding treatment, make sure you are scheduled to see a gynecologic oncologist. If your diagnosis is not clear, but ovarian cancer is suspected, you should still see a gynecologic oncologist. This physician is specifically trained in advanced surgery for gynecologic cancers. If the hospital or cancer center has a Web site, you are encouraged to read through it. You may find information about the doctors that may lead you to a specific doctor who appeals to you. When scheduling your appointment, make sure you confirm that your appointment is with a gynecologic oncologist. Ask the scheduler what you need to bring or if you should arrange for information to be sent to the hospital prior to your visit for advanced review. Unless you are experiencing symptoms (severe pain, vomiting, etc.), you do not have to be seen immediately. However, let the scheduler know that you have or may have ovarian cancer to allow for a prompt appointment.

You will most likely be anxious the day of your appointment. Review the time of the appointment and make sure you bring any records you have. Make sure you have the address of the building and the office number for your appointment. Get directions beforehand and allow yourself time to get there, find parking, get checked into the office (you will probably have to complete some paperwork), and to get settled before you meet with the doctor. It is helpful to bring a family member or friend who can help you take notes during the visit (more about this in the following section).

WHAT TO BRING WITH YOU FOR THAT FIRST CONSULTATION

Ask what you should bring with you to your first visit with the gynecologic oncologist. If you are unsure about what to bring, some general guidelines include any information you have leading up to your diagnosis. This will include any radiographic images (ultrasounds, CAT scans, MRIs) and blood work results. Occasionally, films you have had performed at another institution may not be the right test or may be of poor quality. In this case, you may need additional testing to be done following your visit. It is helpful to check with your insurance company on tests that may require pre-authorization. Additionally, if done at another institution, bring any pathology samples such as the slides from biopsies/aspirations you had performed. It may be helpful to have these sent in advance for the gynecologic oncologist and gynecologic pathologist to review prior to your visit. Typically, the treating physician will keep your films and slides until he/she has had a chance to review everything with specialists (radiologists, pathologists, etc.).

WHO TO BRING WITH YOU TO THE FIRST CONSULTATIVE VISIT

A lot of information will be exchanged at the first visit. Retaining and understanding it may be quite overwhelming. We strongly recommend that you bring a close family member or friend with you to your first visit. Ask this person to write notes so you can remember important points; some patients have even found it helpful to bring a tape recorder. Encourage your guest to ask questions as well.

WHAT ELSE TO BRING FOR THIS INITIAL VISIT

At your initial visit, you will be asked to review your health history. This consists of your medical history (any medical problems you have been diagnosed with) and your surgical history (any procedures/surgeries you have had in the past). Keep a list of your allergies and any medications you are taking, including their dosages. This includes prescription medications and over-the-counter medications, as well as vitamins/herbal remedies. Learn your family medical history, particularly for ovarian and breast cancers.

WHAT QUESTIONS TO ASK DURING YOUR VISIT

A lot of information will be exchanged at this visit. It is good to make a list of questions that you have. Some commonly asked questions by patients in this situation include the following:

1. What type of ovarian cancer do I have?

2. What stage do you suspect that I may be in based on the present information, examination, tests, etc.?

3. Did the pathologist review my slides (if appropriate) and did the interpretation differ from my previous results?

4. What is your philosophy about surgery for ovarian cancer?

5. What procedures do you think will be necessary to successfully debulk the cancer?

6. How many ovarian cancer cases do you perform a year?

7. What is your optimal debulking rate?

8. How soon can my surgery be scheduled?

9. What resources are available for me to help me understand my disease and what to expect during the course of treatment?

10. Does the institution offer an ovarian cancer survivor group?

11. Who do I contact here if I have any questions or problems?

12. Do you have educational materials for me and my family?

13. Who else will be involved in my care?

14. Why would I need chemotherapy after the surgery if all the cancer is removed?

15. If necessary, when will chemotherapy be started?

16. What will my follow-up schedule be like?

17. Who will help in the coordination of my medical care, including scheduling follow-up appointments?

WHAT TESTS NEED TO BE DONE?

Prior to your surgery, it is common to have a computed axial tomography (CAT) scan (or other imaging) done in order to get an idea of whether the cancer has spread to any other organs. This allows the physician to have a better understanding of the extent of the disease and help prepare for surgery.

Blood tests are done in preparation for the operation and are typically standard amongst institutions. These tests are not related to your cancer diagnosis but are important baseline tests to make sure you can tolerate the surgery. They include checking your blood counts, chemistries, in addition to other studies such as a chest X-ray and an electrocardiogram (EKG), which evaluates the heart. A blood test to determine your CA-125 level may be drawn prior to your surgery. The CA-125 is a protein that may be secreted by ovarian cancer cells. It is not mandatory that this test be done before you go to the operating room and this may be drawn following your surgery.

HOW BEST TO CONTACT TEAM MEMBERS

It is important to know the right person to contact. Ask your physician for his or her business card. Make sure you are clear on how your questions and concerns will be addressed, and by whom. It is also important to ask what to do in case of emergency or if something comes up after hours. You may want to ask for the best way to contact the team members: by e-mail (only if you are comfortable with it) or by phone. When you do call, try to ask all of your questions in one call. Some patients find it helpful to write down the questions over time and call when they have a few questions on their list. Of course, in an emergency, you should not wait.

NAVIGATING APPOINTMENTS

Some cancer centers have patient navigators. This term is used to describe a system of assisting patients with their medical care in regards to scheduling appointments and tests, selecting a date for your surgery, and coordinating visits with other services if necessary. This may be some-one in your physician's office or someone who works in the cancer center. In any case, this person should be able to help answer or coordinate anything that you may need in regards to your medical care scheduling.

FINANCIAL IMPLICATIONS OF TREATMENT/
INSURANCE CLEARANCE

Whether you are working outside of the home or not, your diagnosis is probably something for which you were not prepared. In addition to the treatment process, you also have to consider your personal life and the changes you may experience. This may include taking time off work and making financial arrangements for bill payments. If you are working, you should find out how much sick leave you have available and what is your short-term disability coverage. You should also investigate your health insurance policy and know what is your co-payment cost for hospital visits, your prescription coverage plan, and whether you need referrals. Referrals are required by some insurance companies prior to seeing physician specialists, having specific tests performed, getting surgery authorized, and other treatments such as participation in clinical trials. This can be an overwhelming task. Many hospitals have a care coordinator, social worker, or financial assistant available to help assist you. If you need it and it is not offered, ask for help.

If you do not have health insurance, ask for a financial assistant or social worker. There are resources available that may assist you in covering your cancer related expenses. Do not be shy about asking for help. If you do not ask, you may not be given this information. You will find that hospitals often have a wide range of financial support services. Take control of this aspect of your care. This will help you plan your finances, eliminating additional stress for both you and your family.

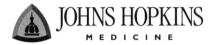

TAKING ACTION—
COMPREHENSIVE TREATMENT
CONSIDERATIONS

The treatment process begins when your diagnosis is first suspected. The purpose of this chapter is to review the different types of treatment and factors that may influence your decision-making process. We review surgery, chemotherapy, and targeted therapy.

SURGICAL TREATMENT

Many women experience anxiety about the surgical removal of the ovaries because these are the organs that secrete the female hormones. After menopause, the ovaries secrete little to no hormonal products. Even prior to menopause, removing the ovaries does not result in a loss of femininity. It is important to talk to family members and your physician about your concerns.

Surgery is the primary modality of treatment for most women. This surgery is often referred to as primary cytoreductive or debulking surgery. The goal of this surgery is to remove as much of the tumor that is present as possible while keeping your safety in mind. There are multiple goals of the surgery. First, surgery will confirm the diagnosis, if not done already. Secondly, when the tumor is large, removing it may provide relief from pain and pressure caused by the disease. Lastly, it has been well established that reducing the largest remaining tumor to one centimeter or less in diameter will result in an improved survival for the patient; this is referred to as optimal cytoreduction. Furthermore, the ability to remove all visible disease, referred to as complete cytoreduction, results in an even better outcome. Optimal cytoreduction is one of the most important factors that influence survival. This brings us back to the initial selection of your surgeon. Having the surgery performed by a gynecologic oncologist results in the chance for optimal or complete cytoreduction that is three times more likely than if performed by another type of surgeon. Therefore, this is one of the most critical choices you will make for your treatment and one you should research thoroughly.

Prior to having the surgery performed, most surgeons will request that you perform a bowel prep. This is a major operation and the incision will most likely be a vertical midline incision starting at the pubic bone and extending above the umbilicus. The surgery typically consists of removing the uterus, cervix, fallopian tubes, and ovaries. Because of the ability of ovarian cancer to spread in the abdomen, other tissues are removed for analysis as well, including the omentum, which is the fatty apron that hangs off of a portion of the large bowel. Ovarian cancer also can spread via lymphatics (a system of vessels that is one of the methods of drainage from the ovaries). The pelvic and para-aortic (by the aorta) lymph nodes therefore may be removed as well. Cancer cells may attach themselves to the lining of the abdominal cavity, called the peritoneum. This may be resected (removed) with a special instrument to destroy the implants. Ovarian cancer also may implant on or invade other organs including the small and large intestines, spleen, liver, or diaphragm (the muscle between the lungs and abdomen), which may require resection or ablation. Remember, the goal is to remove all visible disease, so additional procedures should be done if necessary as long as they can be safely performed.

Surgery is the first step of a lifelong process. You are encouraged to ask questions about which you have concerns. After the date is set for the surgery, you will feel a sense of relief. Focus on the surgery and the recovery process. Take things step by step. At your postoperative visit, when you are ready, you will be given details regarding the next steps.

POST-OPERATIVE CARE

Depending on the extent of your surgery, you may wake up in a hospital room or intensive care unit, which provides additional monitoring after your surgery. You will notice several tubes attached to you that includes at least one intravenous (IV) line in your arm, near your collarbone, or in your neck. These lines are placed so that you can receive fluids and medications through these sites. You also will have a tube delivering oxygen, which can be administered through your nose or by a face mask. Occasionally, particularly when the surgery takes a long period of time or requires extensive procedures, the breathing tube may stay in place overnight or for a couple of days after the surgery. This allows your body to rest while providing additional oxygen to your lungs. If your surgery required a portion of bowel to be resected or a lot of bowel manipulation, you may wake up with a tube in your nose (nasogastric tube). The purpose of this tube is to drain the fluid and air from your stomach. This typically remains in place for several days until your bowel function returns. You may have surgical drains placed. These drains are placed in the abdominal cavity and are brought through the skin. They prevent the accumulation of fluid within the abdomen after the surgery.

As with everything, there are some potential side effects you may experience following the surgery. One of the more common side effects is infections, which may occur in one of many places such as the bladder, the surgical incision site, the IV sites, in the abdominal cavity, or in the bloodstream. The treatment varies based on the site but may include antibiotic treatment or drainage of the infection. Another side effect is bowel dysfunction, which may result in nausea and vomiting. This usually gets better with bowel rest, which includes IV hydration and may require a nasogastric tube as described above. If the bowel dysfunction persists for a long period of time, you may even receive IV nutrition known as parental nutrition. This allows your body to obtain the calories and substances it needs to continue to heal while your appetite is returning or improving. Muscle weakness and fatigue are also common side effects following the surgery and often improve with time and mild activity.

We recommend that you begin physical activity as soon as possible. This allows you to become more comfortable with the incision and allows your muscles to regain strength. In addition, it helps prevent one of the major causes of death after surgery, blood clots in the large vessels of the legs/ pelvis, called deep venous thrombosis, that can break free and travel to the lungs causing a pulmonary embolism. Initially, you will find it a slow process to become accustomed to things you used to do without thinking about before. This includes getting in and out of bed, and even walking. During the beginning stages of the healing process, light lifting (up to 25 pounds) is allowed, but it is wise to avoid any strenuous activity such as running and sit-ups. Many people are afraid of getting the incision wet after the surgery. Though the wound will take several months to heal, rinsing it with soap and water is harmless and a good way to keep the incision clean.

It may take several weeks before you have gained a lot of your strength back. As your energy and strength levels return, you will find yourself doing more and more every day. However, following the surgery, you may need someone at your home to assist you with your recovery. This may include surgical duties such as taking care of drains placed during surgery and postoperative wound care to daily activities such as such as cooking, cleaning, and helping you go up and down a flight of stairs. You will most likely be taking narcotic pain medication after your surgery. These medications provide pain relief but also may make you sleepy and affect your response time. While taking these medications, you should not drive. Even after you are off the narcotic medication, you will want to make sure you can drive safely. This means you will need to be able to move comfortably in addition to driving over bumpy roads and slamming on the brakes. The period of time you need to be able to drive varies on an individual basis. It may be helpful to ask the surgeon about what you can expect in the days and weeks following your surgery.

ADJUVANT TREATMENT AFTER SURGERY

After your surgery, the pathologist will study the surgical tissue and report the degree of spread of the disease. If the disease has spread beyond the ovaries, you will need additional therapy that is given in the form of chemotherapy, which sometimes is referred to as cytotoxic agents. The purpose of the chemotherapy is to sterilize any remaining cancer cells not removed by surgery. The goal is to give the most effective amount of chemotherapy while preventing or minimizing the side effects of the drugs. Though the quality of life is important, adequately treating the disease will result in experiencing some of the side effects. If side effects become too bothersome or dangerous, it may be necessary to adjust your chemotherapy dosages or schedule.

Cancer cells differ from normal cells (noncancerous cells) in several ways. First, cancer cells grow at a much faster rate than the normal cells in the body. Secondly, cancer cells will replicate without limit. This allows them to outgrow the space they started in, resulting in pain or other symptoms.

Chemotherapy works by targeting these differences in the cancer cells. Specifically, it works by killing these cells, stopping them from multiplying, or a combination of the two. Unfortunately, the chemotherapy cannot distinguish the cancerous cells from the fast-growing normal cells of the body. This is what results in the development of side effects, which will be discussed in more detail in Chapter 4.

CHEMOTHERAPY

The first chemotherapy regimen you receive is referred to as front-line or first-line chemotherapy. As mentioned, this is a complement to the surgery and the goal is to achieve a complete clinical remission, which means that there is no evidence of cancer on physical examination, imaging studies, or by the blood test CA-125.

Although slight differences may occur between different institutions, the general standard of care for epithelial ovarian cancer has been well established. In these cases, the chemotherapy course will be comprised of a platinum drug (Paraplatin [carboplatin] or Platinol AQ [cisplatin]) in combination with Taxol (paclitaxel), taxane-based drugs. There are two types of ways to administer the chemotherapy. The first way is given intravenously, that is, through a vein either in the arm or near the collarbone (via an intravenous port). The second way is administered through an intraperitoneal catheter and delivers the chemotherapy directly to the abdominal cavity. This type of chemotherapy is always combined with intravenous administration. The type of administration of the chemotherapy depends on the stage of the disease.

The administration and monitoring of the chemotherapy may vary slightly from hospital to hospital. At our institutions, The Johns Hopkins Hospital and Medical Institutions, we perform the following tests and/or procedures:

Central venous access. As mentioned earlier, some patients choose to have a catheter placed in a central vein (by the collarbone or in the arm), which remains in place for an extended period of time (semipermanent). The catheter may be external, where there is a small tube that comes out through the skin at the level of the collarbone (Hickman catheter) or in the arm (a peripherally inserted central catheter or a PICC line). An internal catheter, such as a Mediport, is where the entire port is underneath the skin. There is a palpable ridge that allows the reservoir of the port to be accessed via a small needle stick. These ports have a lower infection rate than the external catheters; however, both have the advantage of allowing for easy and repetitive venous access. Catheters are not only used for the administration of chemotherapy, but also for other medications, IV fluids, blood transfusions, and used to draw blood samples.

Bloodwork. Prior to the chemotherapy being given, we check some basic laboratory tests. This includes bloodwork such as a complete blood count (CBC), a chemistry panel, and a CA-125 level. This level, when elevated, may be a useful marker for determining if the chemotherapy is effective.

Imaging. Though not always done, you may be asked to have a baseline CAT scan of your abdomen and pelvis. This allows for a comparison of progress during your chemotherapy course. Other films may include a chest X-ray or chest CAT scan.

The chemotherapy will be administered over planned time intervals referred to as the chemotherapy schedule. The first cycle is administered when you can safely tolerate and after you have begun healing from the surgery. This may vary from a relatively short period of time after surgery to up to six to eight weeks following surgery. Following the initial cycle, the schedule is typically set so that you receive your chemotherapy every three weeks. This allows for your body to recover from the previous cycle, particularly in regards to red blood cells, white blood cells, and platelets. You will have blood tests drawn before every cycle and although it is important to stay on schedule, sometimes the body is slower to recover than expected. This may result in a delay of the next chemotherapy cycle for a week or so, or result in a slight decrease in the dosage of the chemotherapy prescribed. Generally this will not impact the effectiveness of the overall treatment.

The goal is to administer six cycles of chemotherapy, making the entire process six to seven months. You will be monitored throughout your course of chemotherapy with physical examinations and CA-125 levels, if indicated. After the third cycle, or the halfway point, the status of your disease and your treatment response will be reassessed using repeat imaging, in addition to bloodwork and the examination, to make sure the cancer is responding to the treatment. If the disease is growing despite the chemotherapy, your regimen may be modified to another drug(s) to find a more effective regimen.

The day prior to the chemotherapy will require preparation. It is recommended that you avoid heavy foods. Also, it is essential that you drink plenty of fluids the day before and the day of chemotherapy. This significantly helps prevent dehydration and may help improve your ability to handle the chemotherapy. You will have anti-nausea medications prescribed for you to take starting the day before the chemotherapy is given. This in addition to other medications, such as a small dose of steroid, work to help you tolerate the chemotherapy and its side effects much better.

The actual time frame when the chemotherapy is administered may vary from an outpatient visit for approximately six hours (IV administration) to an inpatient hospital admission for a day and a half (intraperitoneal administration). You also will receive IV fluids to help with hydration. Some of the medications you take the day of your chemotherapy may be sedating (such as Benadryl [diphenhydramine]), so make sure you have someone to drive you home. We also recommend that you fill any prescriptions you are given prior to leaving the infusion center (this may include medications to help you prepare for the next cycle).

Most side effects occur in the first few days after receiving chemotherapy. Most commonly these include nausea and vomiting or an upset stomach. The anti-nausea medications may reduce these symptoms greatly or even entirely. We recommend that you eat light, bland foods such as carbohydrates (rice, breads, and pastas) for the first few days. The most important thing is that you keep yourself well hydrated with fluids. A more thorough review of the side effects of chemotherapy is provided in the next chapter.

NEOADJUVANT CHEMOTHERAPY

In certain situations, patients may benefit from having chemotherapy before undergoing a surgical procedure. This is referred to as neoadjuvant chemotherapy. The most common reason for this type of therapy is the inability to tolerate surgery due to other medical conditions, or if the patient is "too sick," making the surgery dangerous. Another reason is if the disease is too advanced or has spread to areas in the body that would not allow for optimal cytoreduction. This approach should be taken with caution as it is difficult to predict the extent of disease based on radiographic imaging alone. Often times if a surgeon suspects they will be unable to debulk the disease, he/she will perform a laparoscopic procedure to confirm the suspicion. This allows for the opportunity to perform the surgery if the suspicion was incorrect, or at the least, to obtain a biopsy of the tissue for pathologic assessment. If neoadjuvant chemotherapy is chosen, it may shrink the volume of the tumor; this is confirmed by radiographic imaging studies and the patient's overall health status. This evaluation typically occurs after three to six cycles of neoadjuvant chemotherapy, and if a response is noted, it may make surgery more feasible. This surgery is known as an interval debulking procedure.

HORMONAL THERAPY

On rare occasions, a patient may not be a candidate for or may choose not to take chemotherapy. Certain cancers respond to hormonal therapy. These include breast cancer, endometrial cancer, prostate cancer, and to a lesser degree ovarian cancer. These cancers are hormonally sensitive. By removing the hormone that is able to stimulate the cancer (that feeds the cancer cells), the tumor may respond. In addition to removing the stimulating hormone, the administration of antagonists (chemicals that block the hormone's stimulating response, or oppose that hormone's effects) may help control the disease. A common example of this is Soltamox (tamoxifen), a selective estrogen receptor modulator which blocks estrogen from entering the cancer cells for the treatment of estrogen-receptor positive breast cancer. Well-differentiated ovarian cancers are more likely to respond than those that are not because these tumor cells are more likely to have retained the hormone receptors, thus allowing them to recognize the hormone in the first place. Unfortunately, in regards to ovarian cancer, only a small percentage of women (less than 10%) will respond to hormonal therapy, and usually it is not a long-lasting effect. To determine if a patient has hormone sensitive disease, a tissue specimen or biopsy may be analyzed by the pathologist for the presence of hormone receptors. When a patient is a candidate for hormonal therapy, the target is usually estrogen. Most commonly this is antagonized by progesterones or anti-estrogen medications such as Soltamox. Side effects may include weight gain, headaches, and leg cramps, but these side effects are usually minimal. Because these medications are typically well tolerated, it is usually worth a trial period.

GROWTH-INHIBITING HORMONE THERAPY

As mentioned before, cancer cells may replicate without limit. Finding a way to disrupt these processes may help prevent the growth of ovarian cancers and avoid damage to normal tissues. One current experimental method of approach is to inhibit the formation of new blood vessels to the cancer cells. This prevents the cancerous cells from getting nutrients through the bloodstream and results in cell death. This type of therapy is known as anti-angiogenesis therapy. Other methods of growth inhibiting therapies are currently being studied.

GENE THERAPY

Gene therapy is a complex principle in which the target is not the cell or its resources, but rather the DNA that controls the behavior of the cell. It replaces a damaged piece of DNA with the attempt of making the cell behave normal again. Research has shown that cancer cells have undergone, to some degree, DNA alterations that contribute to its cancerous behavior. Unfortunately, identifying the change is difficult in itself. Furthermore, there may be multiple DNA changes, making the target less clear. Even if the alteration were identified, creating the DNA to replace that change and the vehicle to get it into the cancer cell provides a whole new set of challenges. Scientists are making great progress and the field is beginning to generate a lot of excitement in cancer research.

ANTIBODY THERAPY

Antibody therapy tries to capture the subtle differences between cancer cells and normal cells in the body. Antibodies are proteins that can be created by the immune system or in the laboratory, and function by recognizing antigens (essentially markers on the cell that distinguish them from other cells). When the antibody binds to the antigen, the body's immune system recognizes this complex and disposes of it using a type of white blood cell called a lymphocyte. Finding an antigen specific to cancer cells will allow for an antibody to be made to target these cells. Unfortunately, many normal cells share the same antigens, which limit the effectiveness of this type of therapy. However, promising work continues in the laboratory.

IMMUNOTHERAPY

Immunotherapy also uses the body's defense system to target cancer cells. This type of treatment stimulates an increase in the cancer-fighting immune cells of the body. There are a couple of ways to do this. First, a precursor to your white blood cells can be taken from your bone marrow, grown in the laboratory, and placed back into the body. Another way is to give you a medication that can cause your body to create more white blood cells that then fight the cancer cells. The concept is that the more immune cells there are, the more likely they are to find and clear the cancer cells. Once again, the goal is to target the cancer cells while sparing the normal cells so that side effects are limited. Although both antibody therapy and immunotherapy are logical concepts, there is still a lot of work to be done in these arenas to make them an effective strategy.

INVESTIGATIONAL DRUGS AND CLINICAL TRIALS

Clinical trials are ways to address patients with recurrent diseases who may have run out of conventional options, or ways to determine if a different regimen is better than the currently used medications. The trials are separated into three categories that work in a stepwise fashion.

> *Phase I trials.* These trials determine if and how much of a medication or combination of medications can be given. This essentially tells us the dose at which medicines are tolerated as well as providing insight into the side effects of the medication. At this point, we do not know if the medication will have any benefit for the disease being targeted. Many treatments are deemed to be toxic at this stage and never make it to the next steps.

> *Phase II trials.* These trials are used to determine if a medication is effective or not. This trial only looks at the medication in question and asks—does it work or not? We do not know how it compares to other treatment options available. Now that we know the dosages that are tolerated, as determined by the phase I study, we can try different dosages to see if one dose is better than another. Data on how many people responded will be collected in this phase and also a comparison to other studies that have been previously published (known as historical controls).

Phase III trials. These trials are the "gold standard" of studies. These are systematic studies that evaluate people with the same disease who are being treated by different therapies. If the patient meets the specific criteria, then he or she agrees to participate in the study and is then "randomly" assigned to the treatment group. The word "randomly" means that neither the investigator nor the patient chooses the type of treatment they are to receive. The general design of the trial is one group receives the current standard of treatment and the other group receives the medications being studied. The results of this study typically determine whether the current regimen is the best therapy for the disease or if the new treatment is more effective, creating a new standard of care.

The decision to participate in a clinical trial is an individual one. Make sure you are comfortable with the trial. We have provided a brief list of questions that you may want to consider asking prior to enrolling in the clinical trial.

- What is the purpose of the trial?

- What type of tests and how many visits does the study involve? How does this compare if I weren't enrolled in the study?

- What are the benefits and risks of the medications in the trial?

- What side effects may I expect?

- How long is the study?

- What type of follow-up care is provided?

- Does my insurance company cover the study related costs? Will I be responsible for any additional costs?

- What happens if I cannot complete the study?

- When will the results be reported?

Many patients have benefited from the participation in clinical trials. It is common for the studied therapies to provide patients with better survival results or improved tolerance to medications. In fact, this is how the current standard of care was determined. The role of clinical trials is to continue the evolution of medicine. Therefore, participation in clinical trials may benefit you as well as the tens of thousands of women who are diagnosed with ovarian cancer each year.

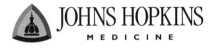

CHAPTER 4

BE PREPARED—
THE SIDE EFFECTS
OF TREATMENT

As you have now become familiar with the surgery and chemotherapy for the treatment of ovarian cancer, it is important to review the possible complications or side effects of these treatments. We discussed common postoperative complications in Chapter 3. In this chapter, we discuss side effects associated with chemotherapy. Just like every patient will respond to treatment differently, every patient will experience different side effects. Some are relatively minor and may be easy to deal with, whereas others may be more difficult. Though the list is long, it is intended to provide you with an overview of the most common side effects of chemotherapy. Ask your doctor who to contact if questions or issues arise.

FATIGUE

The most common complaint of any patient undergoing any type of treatment for cancer is fatigue. Fatigue is a feeling of low energy, weakness and/or tiredness. Unless fatigue is related to anemia (see below), improvement of this symptom may be challenging. Fatigue can occur for many different reasons. First, make sure you are aware of your sleeping habits. Difficulty sleeping at night can affect your energy level and your doctor may be able to prescribe a medication to help you sleep. Spending your energy doing things that are important to you and staying active may actually improve your energy level. Try doing activities with the help of friends and family. Take naps before activities. Pay attention to your energy levels throughout the day and schedule your activities based on how you are feeling. Eat a well rounded diet and drink plenty of fluids.

ANEMIA

Anemia is the term used to describe a low red blood cell (RBC) count. This is measured by checking your hemoglobin, which is an iron-containing protein that carries oxygen to your body. When you are anemic, your body is not getting enough oxygen to function and results in the feeling of tiredness. Severe anemia can be very dangerous, causing headaches, dizziness, shortness of breath, or by affecting the ability of your organs, such as your kidneys and heart, from functioning properly.

Once anemia is diagnosed, there are several treatment options. To help your body produce hemoglobin, you may need to take an iron supplement for an extended period of time. In some cases, medications, such as Epogen (epoetin), Procrit (epoetin), or Aranesp (darbopoetin), may be given to stimulate your bone marrow to make more red blood cells. Sometimes these medications are given right after your chemotherapy to prevent anemia from occurring. If the anemia is severe and needs to be treated immediately, you may require a blood transfusion.

LEUKOPENIA

One of the most dangerous side effects from chemotherapy is a low white blood cell (WBC) count, called leukopenia. This risk usually occurs one to two weeks after you receive your chemotherapy. A low WBC count does not mean you will get an infection, but it does put you at a higher risk of getting an infection. Because this is a known side effect of the chemotherapy, your doctor will be checking levels to monitor the WBC count. You may require antibiotics to help prevent or treat an infection. If your WBCs are too low, your chemotherapy may need to be delayed or adjusted. Just like for anemia, you may be given a medication that can boost your WBCs, such as Neupogen (filgrastim) and Neulasta (pegfilgrastim).

It is important that you try to prevent your risk of infection. Things that you can do include washing your hands frequently—particularly before eating and after using the bathroom—and avoiding large crowds and people who may be sick themselves. Cook and wash foods thoroughly before eating them. Despite the best of care, infections can still occur, so it important for you to be aware of common symptoms related to this including fever, chills, redness or pus around an incision site (surgical or catheter), a cough with fever, or pain/odor with urination. Call your doctor if you experience any of these symptoms.

THROMBOCYTOPENIA

Platelets are also produced by your bone marrow and can be affected by chemotherapy treatment as well. This term is called thrombocytopenia and puts you at increased risk of bleeding. Your platelet count is monitored along with your other blood counts and may require your chemotherapy to be delayed or adjusted if your platelet count is too low. If your platelet counts are low, you are advised to avoid anything that may cause you to bleed and/or bruise. This includes activities like sports (particularly contact sports), shaving, and elective procedures (dental cleaning, biopsies) to name a few. If your platelets are dangerously low, or if you experience bleeding, you may require a platelet transfusion.

NAUSEA/VOMITING

The lining of the gastrointestinal tract is sensitive to chemotherapy as well. Without medications, patients would most likely experience some degree of nausea and vomiting, eventually leading to dehydration and poor nutritional intake. Because we expect nausea and vomiting to occur, the goal is to prevent it. Typically, nausea will occur within the first day of the treatment. Medications, such as the 5-HT antagonist, are prescribed to alleviate this side effect on the day of and a couple of days after chemotherapy treatment. Some patients experience delayed nausea, which occurs a couple of days after the chemotherapy. It may be recommended that you take medication for delayed nausea, even if you feel fine, to prevent it from occurring. Medications used to treat this condition are listed in Table 1.

It is important that you take the prescribed antinausea medication as directed by your nurse or doctor. Remember that even if you are not having any nausea, you should still

Table 1 Common Medications Used for Chemotherapy-Induced Nausea and Vomiting

Class of Drug	Brand (Generic) Name
Phenothiazines	Compazine (prochlorperazine)
	Phenergan (promethazine)
Steroids	Decadron (dexamethasone)
Benzamide	Reglan (metoclopramide)
Antihistamine	Benadryl (diphenhydramine)
5-HT antagonist	Anzemet (dolasetron)
	Kytril (granisetron)
	Zofran (ondansetron)
NK-1 receptor antagonist	Emend (aprepitan)

take the medication to prevent nausea from occurring. Other tips to help prevent or control nausea include avoiding strong smells that can worsen nausea, taking in bland foods and liquids (avoiding spicy, greasy foods, as well as alcohol and caffeine), eating small and frequent meals throughout the day, and drinking plenty of fluids (including popsicles, soups, and sports drinks). Some patients have used acupuncture to help control nausea. Ask about alternative options. Let your doctor know if the antinausea medication is not working for you; you may need to be switched to a different class of drugs. Also, let your doctor know if you are not able to drink/eat anything due to severe nausea, as this may require hospitalization.

CONSTIPATION

Constipation is common. Women who are being treated with narcotic pain medication (after surgery or for continued pain) and those receiving chemotherapy are more prone to its occurrence. Constipation can be avoided by eating a fiber-rich diet, maintaining physical activity, using laxatives and/or stool softeners, and drinking plenty of fluids. Let your doctor know if you have not had a bowel movement in over three days. If you are also experiencing nausea/vomiting, abdominal pain or are unable to pass gas, call your doctor immediately as these may be signs of a bowel obstruction.

DIARRHEA

Some patients experience just the opposite of constipation: diarrhea. This may occur because of surgery on the bowel, specific types of chemotherapy, or be related to infection. Let your doctor know if you are experiencing persistent diarrhea (more than 2–3 days), or if the diarrhea is associated with fevers, is bloody, or is causing you to feel dehydrated. Your doctor may need to prescribe an antidiarrheal agent or check for a bacterial infection (which can be treated by antibiotics); additionally, severe diarrhea may require hospitalization.

NEUROPATHY

Neuropathy is a side effect of specific chemotherapy agents, namely paclitaxel and cisplatin. The nerves that control sensation (responsible for the sense of touch), motor (responsible for movement and tone), and autonomic nerves (responsible for automatic functions such as digestion and bladder function) may be damaged by chemotherapy. Most often, the nerves in the hands and the feet are affected causing a feeling of tingling, numbness, or even burning, referred to as peripheral neuropathy. The symptoms may also include weakness, making it difficult to hold things or even walk, and constipation. Other conditions may worsen neuropathy, such as diabetes, malnutrition, and alcohol abuse.

If you are experiencing neuropathy, wear shoes with good support and use assistance when up and about. Medications that may decrease some of the symptoms of neuropathy include vitamin B supplements, pain medications, steroids, antidepressant medication, and antiseizure drugs. Other options include alternative programs such as acupuncture, massage therapy, or occupational therapy. Though not fatal, neuropathy can be temporary or permanent and may have a huge impact on your daily activities. Let your doctor know if you are experiencing neuropathy as it may require adjustment of your chemotherapy.

COGNITIVE FUNCTION

Women receiving chemotherapy may experience changes in concentration or in memory. This is sometimes referred to as "chemo-brain." The symptoms usually occur during the course of chemotherapy and may last even after the completion of therapy. Try to minimize the impact on yourself by writing down questions, keeping lists of "things to do," and keeping your mind active. If symptoms are severe and include changes in vision, confusion, or seizures, let your doctor know immediately.

ALOPECIA

The chemotherapy used to treat ovarian cancer will cause you to lose your hair. This is because chemotherapy targets rapidly growing cells in our bodies such as cancer, but also normal cells such as hair follicles. This mostly affects the hair on your head, but may also affect your eyebrows and eyelids. Though it is not dangerous, hair loss (the medical term is alopecia) can be emotionally difficult to deal with because it affects our self-image. The hair loss begins to occur a couple weeks after the first treatment. Many patients choose to get a wig prior to having the hair loss, which helps them make the transition smoothly. Most cancer centers will have a salon/boutique that is tailored for cancer patients and will help find a good fit for you. Insurance companies may cover the cost of a wig (also known as a cranial prosthesis), so check your policy. If you choose not wear a wig, there are other options such as hats, scarves, and make-up that may help you adjust. In addition, many patients will get their hair cut short, or even shave their head prior to losing it. This lets you take control of the situation and may even make you feel better.

PALMAR-PLANTAR ERYTHRODYSESTHESIA (HAND-FOOT SYNDROME)

Women receiving specific types of chemotherapy, usually for recurrent disease may develop a condition called palmar-plantar erythrodysesthesia, also known as hand-foot syndrome. Chemotherapy agents that may cause this reaction are pegylated liposomal Doxil (doxorubicin), Taxotere (docetaxel), and Cytoxan (cyclophosphamide) to name a few. This condition includes a wide range of symptoms that typically present on the palms of the hands and soles of the feet, such as a tingling sensation, skin discoloration (pink or red color), swelling, and blistering of the skin. This condition may require comfort measures such as lotions and protective barriers (gloves, socks) or even decreasing or discontinuing the dose of chemotherapy.

SEXUAL DYSFUNCTION

Sexual dysfunction may occur after surgery and during and following treatment with chemotherapy. This may be a result of a decreased libido secondary to your self-image as your body changes—scars, hair loss, weight changes—or due to side effects of the treatment such as fatigue. Most women don't feel comfortable discussing this with their doctor, although it might be very important to you. Try different levels of intimacy until you are comfortable. You may need to use vaginal lubricants to help with vaginal dryness. We also encourage you to talk to your partner, which can help with becoming more comfortable with one another.

From the day of surgery to the completion of chemotherapy is a long and tough road; however, preparing for what lies ahead is crucial. Though we have reviewed the more common side effects, never hesitate to ask your doctor if you are experiencing anything unusual. Taking an active part in your own care and being aware of how to recognize, or even manage, side effects when they occur will make the course a little smoother.

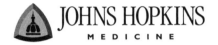

CHAPTER 5

STRAIGHT TALK— COMMUNICATION WITH FAMILY, FRIENDS, AND COWORKERS

Your world probably changed when you were diagnosed with ovarian cancer. It will also directly or indirectly affect those around you, including family members, friends, coworkers, and acquaintances. It is important for you to decide not only who you want to tell, but what you want to tell them. This step can be very challenging. Some women will want to keep their diagnosis very quiet, so as to not burden anyone else or to maintain their own privacy. Most patients will want to tell people closest to them. Letting people know that you are being treated for ovarian cancer can give you a strong support system that will provide you with help in coordinating your care, updating others on your status (if desired), and helping you with your everyday well-being.

This is the time for you and people close to you to take charge of your situation. Select a person (or people) to attend your appointments with you. Make a list of questions to ask regarding your treatment and what to expect. Write down the answers (or have your designated person write them down). This will make your appointments more focused and help you to recall answers later. You should note that these answers may change over time as your disease is treated or as new medications/treatments options are discovered. Ask your doctor if there have been updates every once in awhile and do your own research. Web sites such as **http://www.cancer.gov** or **http://www.nih.gov** can provide information that is helpful for you and those close to you.

Once you have selected who you want to let know about your condition, you should also think about what you want to tell them. Because of the physical effects that the treatment may have on you, such as hair loss and some possible limitations on your energy/activity level (see Chapter 4), people around you may become aware of the situation surrounding you. Start with those closest to you—they can help you tell others when the time is right.

Telling family members is difficult. The emotional effect it has on them may be as strong as it was on you. Additionally, it presents itself as a "crisis" and can be quite stressful. This may even create friction between family members and yourself, or among each other. It is important that you have a support system that is functional, and seeking counseling for family members who are having a difficult time dealing with your treatment may be a helpful option. Don't let family members take over your care; their roles should be that of your advocates and your supporters. Make sure each family member understands his/her role. It may even be helpful to set up one contact person to update everyone else regarding your care, such as through a group e-mail. This can provide the same information to the people you want to share it with in a timely fashion.

Telling your children is also an important issue that you may need to address, whether they are very young or older. Be honest with your children. Let them know about your diagnosis and what type of treatment you will be receiving. You may want to wait until you have discussed the treatment plan with your doctor, but it will help them to cope with the process if they know what to expect (such as hair loss, nausea, fatigue, and frequent appointments). Make sure you also understand their knowledge of cancer. Some children may think that cancer means death. Be reassuring. Cater to the age level of your children and speak their language.

Children and other family members may be affected by your diagnosis if they think they are at increased risk of developing ovarian cancer, too. Provide them with information (if they are old enough) and involve them in the process. It will help them learn about the disease, treatments, and the overall process. Ask your doctor if it is appropriate for you to see a genetic counselor. If so, consider taking family members along who may also benefit from meeting with the genetic counselor and hearing the discussion. This can give your family more information and even make you closer as you deal with the disease.

The decision is yours, but you may want to notify coworkers and employers of your situation to prepare for time off of work as well. You don't have to tell your diagnosis to your employer. There are laws, such as the American Disabilities Act, that provides you with some job security if you do need time off for medical care.

One potential benefit of telling your friends, family, and coworkers is the support that you will receive. It is the natural response to feel compassion for someone undergoing a difficult time in their lives. Your condition may increase awareness of the disease among family, friends, and coworkers and may even inspire them to raise awareness in the community or have a fundraiser for cancer societies, you, and your family. Many people will ask how they can help you during this time. You will have so many things to focus on that this should be a welcomed invitation. Ask for help with meal preparation, babysitting, driving you to appointments or children to their events, and helping with everyday errands and chores, to name a few. Sometimes just asking them to spend time with you can be very helpful.

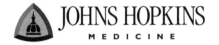

CHAPTER 6

MAINTAINING BALANCE—
WORK AND LIFE DURING
TREATMENT

HELPFUL HINTS ON HOW TO PLAN CARE AND
MINIMIZE DISRUPTIONS IN YOUR LIFE

Being diagnosed with cancer in itself is a disruption. However, it is important that you try to maintain a normal schedule—as much as possible—even during your treatments. Because you will have multiple doctor appointments and "bad" days after chemotherapy, this will require help from others. Understandably, we often have a hard time asking, or even accepting, help from our friends, family, and others. It is important to realize that the treatment you are undergoing will change your routine. Asking for assistance might help you until you are more comfortable with the hectic nature of your schedule.

It is important to include your family in your schedule and the typical course after your treatments are given. Talk to loved ones, particularly children, about how your treatment will affect you and how it might even affect them. Allow your family to understand what you are going through and how it may be necessary for them to help with old and new responsibilities during this time.

The most preparation will be in regards to your surgery and recovery period. Prior to your surgery, you should have a basic understanding of what procedure is going to be done and what you may need to take care of afterwards. This includes postoperative drain care or maintenance of an intravenous or intraperitoneal port. The recovery period after surgery varies based on your overall health status prior to the surgery as well as on the extent of the procedure(s) performed. Ask your surgeon what the average inpatient hospital stay is and how long you will need assistance when you are discharged. Remember, you will need assistance with routine activities and initially, it is recommended that you do not drive for a period of time after your surgery due to the use of pain medications as well as other reasons.

The recovery period is also a time when your incision will be healing. Ask your surgical team what other restrictions you are under, such as lifting heavy objects or strenuous exercise. Most surgeons will encourage you to walk and try to resume a normal schedule as soon as possible.

In order to help stay organized, try to keep a calendar of your appointments and chemotherapy schedule. This will let you know what days you have lab draws, doctor visits, etc. Additionally, it will help you become aware of what days you need to take it easy and what days are typically your strong days. Some patients prefer to have chemotherapy early in the week so that they can have more energy on the weekends, and others like to have chemotherapy late in the week to allow for recovery time over the weekend. Think about what is important in your life and try to set your schedule accordingly. You may have to take other people's schedules into consideration as well; for instance, if someone is driving you to your appointments. Remember, chemotherapy may require several hours of the day, so you may want company during that time.

When you return to work is an individual decision. You have to be ready. Even after surgery your treatment course is in its early stage. If chemotherapy is recommended for you, you will most likely have office visits and lab appointments multiple times in one month. Furthermore, you will have to see how you feel after the chemotherapy to determine how you should set your schedule, both social and work related. However, some women find continuing work allows them to get back to their normal life. It may provide you with a feeling of motivation and distract you from thinking about your cancer diagnosis or treatments. You may find your workplace to be a very supportive environment. There may be times when you will have to arrive late or leave early to keep your appointments or receive treatment. Try to let your employer and coworkers know if you think it will make it easier for you and prevent disruptions in your work.

Infection is always a concern in patients whose white blood cells are affected by the chemotherapy (see page 39). When your white blood count is low, it puts you at higher risk for infection, such as colds or other types of infections. Keep in mind that being in places where you are at increased risk of infection, such as working with young children, hospitals, and crowded places, may require you to take off a little more time to prevent getting an infection during your chemotherapy. Talk to your chemotherapy nurse about when this is most likely to occur and plan accordingly. Some patients will wear a mask over their nose and mouth to prevent breathing any germs, which can significantly decrease the risk. If one of your caretakers is sick, this may even be recommended in your home environment.

Make sure hand washing is a ritual in your household, both yourself and your visitors. Prevent infection when possible. For instance, keep up on your dental health (preferable if done prior to the start of chemotherapy), and it may help to have the influenza (flu) vaccine prior to your chemotherapy if offered at that time. You can maintain your nutritional strength by eating a well balanced diet including fruits and vegetables. Make sure that all fruits and vegetables are washed thoroughly prior to eating them; and that all other foods, including meats, are cooked thoroughly.

Traveling is not off limits during your treatment regimens, but several considerations should be made. First, if traveling by air or bus, consider wearing a mask to reduce the risk of infection. Know of local hospitals in the area you are staying in case of emergency and even consider having your updated records (or a medical summary) with you. Always keep the contact information of your cancer team available in case it is needed.

After you receive chemotherapy, plan on taking it easy for the next day or so. Though medications should be prescribed to prevent nausea, you may still experience it. This typically occurs in the first few days after chemotherapy is given. Make sure you are in a setting that allows you to rest and keep yourself well hydrated. Once you have completed one cycle of chemotherapy, you may be better able to predict what to expect with the next treatments.

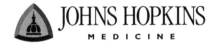

CHAPTER 7

JOHNS HOPKINS
MEDICINE

SURVIVING OVARIAN CANCER— RE-ENGAGING IN MIND AND BODY HEALTH AFTER TREATMENT

SURVIVORSHIP

The term survivorship means different things to different people. Some patients consider it to apply to the minute they were diagnosed and start treatment. Others think of themselves as a survivor after they complete treatment. In general, survivorship is so much more than a definition. It relates to your mental and physical well-being after diagnosis. In the United States, there are approximately 175,000 women living with or a history of ovarian cancer. Each one probably has a different perspective on survivorship. That said, each woman may handle her time differently. By the time you define yourself as a survivor, you too may find that you have a different perspective on many of life's issues.

Some patients consider the diagnosis of cancer to be a "wake-up call." They realize they may need to shift their priorities to enjoy life. This may mean spending more time with family, traveling, or doing things that bring happiness to themselves and others. Patients also focus on maintaining a healthy lifestyle and join exercise or wellness programs. Some patients feel empowered and join groups to help educate and support women who are undergoing treatment for or are survivors of ovarian cancer. One valuable organization is the National Ovarian Cancer Coalition (**http://www.ovarian.org**).

Unfortunately, some patients allow the cancer to consume their lives, even if they are disease-free. They may feel upset with themselves, their doctors, their family, or even their religion for letting them down. Sometimes patients become so involved in their cancer care that when they are done, they actually feel lost, like they don't know what to do next. They are constantly thinking about the disease recurring and allow those thoughts to interfere with many of their daily activities, such as sleeping. Though these patients are living, they are not surviving. Of course, it is common for every patient to have these thoughts or feelings at some time, but it is important to prevent it from taking over every moment. Remember, most cancer centers offer support for survivors of cancer and their spouses and families. Participating in a support group may help you to maintain or regain balance in your life.

COUNSELING

Most people experience a feeling of fatigue or weakness after their cancer treatment. This will definitely affect your energy and activity levels. However, if you feel like you are having a harder time adjusting, you may consider seeing a counselor. Counseling may provide an avenue for discussing issues that are preventing you from getting back to a healthy physical and emotional state. Counseling also provides resources that can help you to cope with any problems you may be experiencing. Another valuable resource, as mentioned earlier, includes participating in ovarian cancer support groups or organizations. Studies have shown that women who participate in a support group have a higher quality of life and live longer than those who do not.

MANAGING LONG-TERM SIDE EFFECTS

In Chapter 4, we discussed some of the more common side effects to expect. Unfortunately, it is common for some of these side effects of treatment to linger even after the cancer is gone. Fatigue is the most common side effect after undergoing any type of cancer treatment. It may persist for months or even years after your treatment, so be prepared. Depending on your status before the surgery, some women may experience surgical menopause. This consists of a set of symptoms, most notably hot flashes, difficulty concentrating, irritability, and vaginal dryness. Most patients will not be candidates for replacement estrogen (the hormone that is lacking that results in these symptoms). Treating these symptoms individually may be helpful. This may include the use of an antidepressant, vaginal lubricants, etc. Also, make sure you protect your bones with vitamin D and calcium, as estrogen helps maintain bone strength. Some patients may develop neuropathy during their treatment. Give your body some more time to heal and in the meanwhile, wear good support shoes and be cautious when handling objects. There are medications that can help minimize the symptoms of neuropathy, but once again, time is key. Share your symptoms with your doctor if symptoms worsen after your treatment and continue to let friends and family help you.

LIVING A HEALTHIER LIFESTYLE

Now that you are a survivor, it is important that you take charge of your overall health. This will not only make you stronger, but may even improve your emotional health. There are many ways to accomplish this. Below are a few suggestions to help you lead a healthier life.

DIET

Everyone should be mindful of their eating habits, regardless. However, now that you have been diagnosed with ovarian cancer, the matter takes on even more importance. Eating a well-balanced diet, maintaining a healthy weight, and getting plenty of exercise will help you to feel better about yourself and life as a whole. Your immune system is boosted, you will sleep better, and feel stronger.

Surviving ovarian cancer is just part of the battle. Eating well reduces your risk for other deadly conditions such as heart disease (the most common cause of death in women), diabetes, and colon cancer—just to name a few. Eating a diet high in fiber, low in fats, and rich in vitamins and minerals is key to good nutritional health. Of course, sweets in moderation are also good for your sense of well-being.

WEIGHT

Along with a healthy diet comes the ability to maintain a healthy weight. If you are overweight, returning to a normal weight is critical. However, doing it in a safe and effective manner is the key to good health. There are many ways to lose weight. You may see advertisements for diet pills and other fads, but these are usually ineffective and sometimes dangerous diets, so avoid these methods. The best way is to incorporate a healthy diet and exercise, and make them permanent parts of your routine. Encouraging your family and/or friends to join you in your quest to lose weight will help you stay on target.

EXERCISE

As mentioned earlier, exercise is an important part of healthy living. If this is a new part of your life, start slow and work up to a good pace. You may need to consult your doctor if you have other health issues to make sure you choose an exercise program that is safe for you. A brisk walk for half an hour three to five times a week is a good start. In addition, add some strength training, starting with three- or five-pound weights, to your exercise regimen. Not only does weight lifting help build muscle, but it also helps maintain bone strength. Once again, have family and friends join you to keep you on pace and make it more enjoyable.

In addition to a traditional exercise regimen, you could engage in different types of exercise programs, such as yoga and tai chi. Yoga is a form of exercise that creates a union (*yoga* is the Sanskrit word for union) of the mind, body, and spirit. The exercises combine breathing techniques and moving mindfully from one body posture to another to create a balance between strength and flexibility. Yoga can create a sense of well-being and relaxation. Classes with an instructor are offered in many cities, but yoga can easily be learned through watching programs offered on television and DVDs or in books, so you can do them at home. Another exercise program that incorporates the mind–body philosophy is tai chi. This program uses martial arts movements, together with breathing and focus to create a sense of relaxation.

Many other activities can help you to stay fit (in both mind and body), including art therapy, aromatherapy, meditation, and massage therapy, just to name a few. Find out what programs are offered near you and try them out to see what helps you obtain a sense of well-being.

AVOID BAD HABITS

Along with your healthy diet and exercise regimen, try to avoid dangerous habits. This includes smoking, even second-hand smoke. Encourage friends and family to quit smoking or refrain from smoking when they are around you. Minimize your alcohol intake, too. If you choose to drink, try to limit yourself to one drink per day.

STRESS

No matter where you are in the treatment process, whether just starting, in the idle, or finishing, undoubtedly you will be faced with a lot of stress. This may be related to your cancer and cancer care, or to the daily stressors of life—family issues, financial issues, etc. How well you are able to cope with and respond to the stress is important. Stress not only contributes to body aches and pains, it also weakens the immune system, which is important for fighting cancer and infections. Although stress is a normal part of everyday life, how you deal with the stress is critical. Some patients learn meditation or other relaxing techniques to reduce stress. Most importantly, most cancer patients learn to let the little things go. This allows you to focus on life's more important issues. Keep things in perspective. Remember, you are a cancer survivor.

SETTING NEW GOALS

The entire process to date has probably changed almost every facet of your life. This is an excellent time to reassess your life. Issues that arise include whether you want to continue working, and if so, work full-time or part-time. You must also consider how you want to spend time with your family and friends. Are you going to pick up new hobbies, things you've always wanted to do? Is this the time to change and devote more attention towards creating a healthier lifestyle? Do you want to educate your community about ovarian cancer and your experience?

Whatever you decide, this is the time to set short-term and long-term goals. Consider reaching out to support groups to find women who have been through a similar situation as you. You may find new friendships as well as resources to help you restart your life. Some patients report that keeping a diary is beneficial. Most importantly, keep the lines of communication open. Your family and friends may expect things to return to "normal," or how things were before your diagnosis. This may not be possible, which will require adjustments on everyone's part. Share your goals with those around you to help them to understand and to support you in the process of reaching those goals.

SEEING THE WORLD THROUGH DIFFERENT EYES

The process that you just went through most likely has changed your life and deeply affected those closest to you. You may have a new perspective on things and realize how precious life really is. This is the time for you to not only focus on yourself and your own health, but that of your family and friends as well. You may want to stay active. This may mean with your loved ones, your job, or something new such as volunteering in hospitals/chemotherapy units or with ovarian cancer organizations. Many patients have said that helping a fellow ovarian cancer patient through the process they just completed is not only beneficial to the new patient, but provides them with a sense of empowerment. Even providing education to increase ovarian cancer awareness in your community (schools, churches, and other groups) can result in saving lives by inspiring women to be evaluated sooner and receiving care by the appropriate team. Giving back is very rewarding and may help you emotionally as well. This takes time though, so make sure you have recovered from your own experience and feel ready to get back out there.

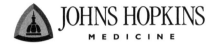

CHAPTER 8

MANAGING RISK—WHAT IF MY CANCER COMES BACK?

D espite a good response to ovarian cancer, the risk of recurrence is one of the biggest fears in women with ovarian cancer. Unfortunately, many women are asked to deal with this issue. It is reported that approximately 60% of women with ovarian cancer will experience a recurrence of their disease. We have not yet identified ways to predict which patients are more likely to experience a recurrence. Knowing what to look for therefore is an important part of your follow-up care.

When a recurrence is diagnosed, it is typically harder to cure. Additionally, the management approach to recurrent disease will vary between a range of treatment options. That is, there is no one set way to deal with recurrent disease. Though there are more commonly followed principles, there are several reasons for the lack of a single approach. First, your treatment will be affected by the time from your original diagnosis to your recurrence. Second, the location where your disease recurs and the extent the abnormal cells have grown will impact your treatment plan. Third, what your body can tolerate will have significant impact on which treatment plan you receive. Another important factor that may arise includes your own individual wishes, which may alter a treatment plan entirely.

PREVENTION AND MONITORING FOR RECURRENCE

For those of you who have undergone surgery and/or chemotherapy, most likely you will be followed closely by your gynecologic oncologist with frequent pelvic examinations and, if an appropriate marker for you, a CA-125 blood test. You may undergo routine imaging studies to look for disease that is not evident on examination. These methods may allow for earlier detection of recurrent disease, although new ways to identify recurrence as early as possible is a hot area of research. New blood tests, just like the CA-125 level, are being developed with the hopes that recurrences will be detected sooner allowing therapy to be more effective. These tests, such as Ovacheck and HE4, use a protein(s) that is specific to ovarian cancer cells, and are used not only to detect early recurrence but also a response to treatment. Though work is ongoing, this area of research shows a lot of promise.

Despite the tests you undergo, it is important to inform your doctor if you develop new symptoms (which often are similar to the original symptoms). If a recurrence is suspected because you have an abnormal exam, scan, or elevated CA-125 level, you may undergo additional imaging studies to help identify the presence or absence of disease. If a mass is found, you may be asked to undergo a needle biopsy in order to confirm that the lesion is recurrent ovarian cancer.

Once a diagnosis of recurrence is made, the decision-making process begins again. Options for management may include surgery. Sometimes surgery is not an option and treatment may include chemotherapy, hormonal therapy, participation in a clinical trial, radiation treatment, or simply observation. Occasionally, the patient may not be able to tolerate any more treatments or chooses not to; in these cases, we provide supportive and comfort care. Let's review the decision-making process and each of the options individually.

One of the most important factors when determining how to treat recurrent disease is by evaluating the amount of time that has passed since the completion of the first course of chemotherapy. This is the time when you would be deemed disease-free (otherwise, you would receive more chemotherapy and not fall into this category). If the disease recurs in a short time interval, typically defined as six months or less, it is more difficult to treat the tumor. This is because the first and most effective chemotherapy (a platinum- and taxane-based regimen) for ovarian cancer had a short-lived effect on the cancer. Although using different agents may provide some patients with a good response to treatment, these patients are usually the exception and not the rule. The most commonly used drugs for recurrent disease are mentioned a little later in this chapter.

TREATMENT OPTIONS

SURGERY

Occasionally, patients will be candidates for a second surgery with the goal of removing the recurrent tumors. This is known as secondary cytoreductive surgery or tumor reductive surgery. The same goals apply to this procedure as to the initial surgical procedure: to remove all visible disease, or to leave as small of a volume as possible. Achievement of these goals is more likely to result in a longer survival time. If the disease is unable to be surgically resected to a volume less than 1 cm, then the benefits of surgery are limited in regards to your survival. If resection of the disease is not possible, the risks and recovery required from surgery make this an unfavorable choice. Most importantly, patients must realize that undergoing surgery is associated with major complications. Even though a patient may be an ideal candidate for surgery in regards to her tumor, the surgeon may believe the risk of complications are too high and offer other therapies.

Patients who are most likely to benefit from secondary cytoreductive surgery are those with a high level of function, limited areas of disease (that is, isolated or restricted to a few tumor masses in areas that can be safely removed), and an adequate time interval from the completion of the initial therapy. Once again, if the disease recurs in the six-month time frame (as described above), surgery is usually not an option, though exceptions may occur.

CHEMOTHERAPY

Whether or not surgery is a good choice for you, almost all women will receive some form of chemotherapy, known as second-line chemotherapy. The choice of chemotherapy is often determined on an individual basis using certain facts. The first fact evaluated is typically the time interval from the completion of the first-line chemotherapy. If this time frame is less than six months, then the chemotherapy used is different from the original regimen because the tumor is less likely to respond to those drugs. The agents used most commonly include Doxil or Hycamtin (topotecan), but may include other drugs or clinical trials (such as those using investigational drugs). If the time frame exceeds six months, the use of the primary agents is more likely to have a response. This may be as originally administered (a platinum and taxane) or with other drugs to enhance the effectiveness (such as a platinum and Gemzar [gemcitabine]).

Another important point to consider is the drugs' toxicities, including those experienced from the first regimen and the potential toxicities from the proposed regimen. As you now know, every chemotherapy agent is associated with side effects. For example, if someone experienced significant neuropathy or renal dysfunction, the oncologist may prefer one drug over another to reduce the risk of worsening any of these side effects. Along these same lines, if a patient is not fully functioning, the chemotherapy agent or dose may be adjusted to make the treatment more tolerable while still having effect on the tumor.

Several for-profit laboratories currently are conducting tests on tumors removed from patients at the time of secondary cytoreductive surgery to determine which chemotherapy agents are most likely to work, or not work, against the tumor. Though these tests are not perfect, research has supported the use of the tests to improve treatment of the cancer. Another benefit is that the tests may indirectly reduce side effects by eliminating the treatment with drugs that are not likely to be beneficial. Ask your doctor about these tests if you are scheduled to secondary cytoreductive surgery.

CLINICAL TRIALS

Often, when the disease recurs (sometimes even in the primary setting), clinical trials may be opened in your local hospital that focus on studying new drugs, new combinations of drugs, new schedules, or new dosages of agents with the goal of improving overall patient survival. In order to determine the best treatments, one arm of the study is compared to another arm. For example, a new drug that has shown promise in ovarian cancer is given to some patients and the results are compared to those from a different group of patients given a drug with known activity against ovarian cancer. The study results determine which drug is superior (both in activity and side effects) and often leads to a new treatment regimen. We strongly recommend participation in clinical trials because the opportunity to try new drugs/treatments is the basis of discovering the latest breakthrough in cancer treatment. Though one of the risks of clinical trials is that the treatment will not work, clinical trials are designed for the best interest of the patient—with tests for detecting tumor growth/response—and if a drug does not work, the patient is taken off of the trial. Not everyone will qualify for a clinical trial, so ask your doctor if any are available.

RADIATION THERAPY

Radiation has no role in first-line therapy for women with ovarian cancer. It may, however, have a limited role in women with recurrent disease. It is typically used in the setting of an isolated recurrence that has been resected, or if there is local unresectable disease that can cause considerable concern or symptoms, such as disease that has spread to the bone, brain, lungs, etc.

HORMONAL TREATMENT

This class of therapy encompasses several groups of drugs, which will be described briefly below. The first group are the progesterones, which in addition to estrogen, are the major hormones produced in the ovary. Though these medications have shown a beneficial response in patients with endometrial cancer, the data in ovarian cancer are not as strong. However, these medications are used for another property—stimulating the appetite, resulting in weight gain—in patients who require it due to poor nutrition from to the cancer treatments or the cancer itself.

The second group is known as selective estrogen receptor modulators (SERMs) and includes drugs like Soltamox and Evista (raloxifene), which essentially block estrogen from the cells. These drugs have a modest response rate in ovarian cancer and do not have major toxicities. SERMs may provide some control in women in whom other therapy is not well tolerated.

The next group is known as aromatase inhibitors (Arimidex [anastrozole], Femara [letrozole], etc.), which also block estrogen. These drugs probably have a response rate similar to the SERMs as well as a favorable toxicity profile.

The last group of drugs in this category is the antigonadotropins. These drugs block the production of gonadotropins, the hormones that stimulate the ovaries to produce hormones. Though the ovaries most likely have been removed, it has been shown that ovarian cancer cells have gonadotropin receptors and that these drugs may provide a low response rate in some patients. Though this class of drugs shows some promise, more research needs to be performed to demonstrate the true activity of these drugs in the recurrent setting of ovarian cancer.

OBSERVATION

Occasionally patients with ovarian cancer may have a recurrence but not require or be fit for additional treatment. If a patient has a slow growing tumor (low grade) that is asymptomatic, the "watch and wait" treatment strategy may be used. This method is useful when the risks of the therapy (chemotherapy, surgery, etc.) are greater than the benefits. Each treatment approach has its own goals and occasionally observation is the most effective treatment plan. This is a much different approach than when the cancer is no longer curable or controllable (discussed in detail in Chapter 9).

OTHER OPTIONS

A lot of attention has focused on "natural" or "herbal" remedies, specifically medications. Be careful when considering this option. There is quite a bit of literature on these products, but most of it is in the form of advertisements (even though it doesn't look like it) or created without much—or any—research to support the health claims. Additionally, these products are often referred to as vitamins or nutritional supplements, and not medications. Many of these products are not FDA approved and may play on the "will try anything" mentality of some cancer patients. These methods are often quite expensive and sometimes actually may be dangerous. Do your own research (or ask a medical professional) before experimenting. Let your doctor know if you do take anything because it may interfere with your other treatments.

Though this chapter provides a review of the most commonly used therapies for recurrent ovarian cancer, research is continually underway to determine newer and more effective options. Remember, treatment is individualized and dependent on several factors that may use one or a combination of the treatment regimens listed above. The goal is to control the disease without compromising your safety and quality of life.

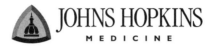

CHAPTER 9

My Cancer Isn't Curable— What Now?

UNDERSTANDING THE GOALS OF TREATMENT FOR METASTATIC DISEASE

Ovarian cancer is often found at advanced stages of the disease. In many cases, chemotherapy can provide a good clinical response. But when the disease becomes resistant to chemotherapy or the body cannot handle the treatment due to side effects, the focus shifts from curing the disease to keeping the disease in control. Of course, it is natural to want all of the cancer out of your body. Unfortunately, our treatment choices may not offer such an option. The goal of treatment is now control and this may be done by stabilizing the disease with therapy and finding a peaceful co-existence for you and the cancer. This hopefully will allow you to maintain a good quality of life (detailed later in this chapter) with little or no awareness of the cancer itself.

Sometimes the treatment may range from chemotherapy, with side effects, to gentler medications such as hormonal therapy, which is generally well tolerated. Think of the treatment as one for a lifelong condition—such as maintaining blood pressure or treating diabetes. Without treatment the diseases would take over and wreak havoc on your body, causing strokes, blindness, heart attacks, etc. With treatment, the disease is still there but less likely to cause problems. The same applies to ovarian cancer treatment in this setting. The treatment doesn't rid your body of the cancer but attempts to prevent it from affecting your body in a negative way. In essence, your ovarian cancer is a chronic condition and needs to be treated as such.

SETTING SHORT-TERM GOALS

Though not always easy, this is the time to be realistic. You may have to think of your life in a set of short-term blocks. Instead of setting goals for ten or even five years from now, think of starting with even briefer time intervals, or short-term goals. A lot of your outcome will be based on how you respond to chemotherapy, whether it is the first round of chemotherapy or the fourth. Start with goals that cover a one-year time frame.

Of course, there are women who have been cured from advanced disease, but we cannot predict who will fall into this group and who will not. It is good, therefore, to understand the disease and its natural course. Talk to your doctor about what to expect. Think positively, but don't lose sight of reality. Making long-term plans may be okay, but do what is most important to you in the present. You may be alive in three years, but remember that the chemotherapy and other treatments may not allow you to be as active as you once were. See how your body, and even your mind, responds to treatments. Be aware of checkpoints in your care. Ask your physician when you will have repeat tests/images to see if the treatment is working. Use these milestones to set your next set of short-term goals.

QUALITY OF LIFE VERSUS QUANTITY OF LIFE

Regardless of disease status, quality of life should always be at the forefront of your thoughts. This means that living a miserable life filled with pain to the age of 100 is by far less desirable than living a shorter life pain-free and happy. There should always be an emphasis on not just quantity of life—keeping you alive—but on quality of life, making sure you enjoy the days you are alive. Along with your short-term goals, think of where you want to be, what you want to do, and with whom you want to spend the time you have left.

Issues that affect quality of life are many and often aren't apparent to your medical providers. For instance, if you are experiencing pain, let your physician know. They may be able to provide you with pain medication or other treatments to help reduce this pain. This is one of the priorities in providing you with quality of life. Strategies may include radiation to shrink a tumor that is compressing a nerve, minor surgery to bypass an obstruction in your bowels or alleviate chronic nausea, or support services that may help you emotionally. Some patients fear that telling the doctor these symptoms may mean the end of treatment. Though this may be true in some cases, it may also mean that another treatment would be better, or that the treatment itself is causing more problems than benefits. You are encouraged to let your team of medical providers know if you are not comfortable. Very often something can be done to improve your symptoms without compromising your time. It is up to you to find the balance between quality of life and quantity of life.

WHEN SHOULD I STOP TREATMENT?

This question must be answered on an individual basis. There is no easy answer for this question, nor is the answer the final one. For instance, you may choose to stop for a period of time and then choose to begin again—because you are ready, or because there is a new treatment available. However, it is critical that you and your physician have an open meeting about the course of your disease. Encourage your family to be part of the discussion as well. Generally, treatment is a reasonable option as long as you are demonstrating a response—decrease in tumor volume or stabilization of the disease—and you are not experiencing intolerable side effects. If the treatment isn't helping, it could be more harmful to continue it than to stop it. Try to be as prepared as possible. Be aware of your response to treatment and ask your doctor to be honest with you on what the future holds. This is not easy for your physician either but can make the transition smoother in the long run. Ask what future options are, including clinical trials, if the current treatment you are on does not work.

Once all options are used, you should think about your condition being incurable. Knowing a realistic timeline may help you keep your life in order as well. Plan for your personal matters to be taken care of, such as having a living will or advance directives (which states clearly what you want done, or what you don't want done when death is approaching), choosing a power of attorney (when you designate someone to make healthcare decisions for you if you are unable to do so for yourself), and making important financial arrangements as well as the many other issues that you believe need to be addressed. Though death can happen to anyone at any time, you have the opportunity to be better prepared. Be specific about what you want done. Does this include cardiopulmonary resuscitation (CPR), which may include placing you on a ventilator to help you breathe, performing chest compression, and giving medications to keep your heart pumping? It is important for you to understand your own choices and share that information with your family and your physician, so they can honor your wishes.

HOSPICE/PALLIATIVE CARE

There comes a point in the care of patients with cancer when the side effects of the medications/treatment become greater than the benefit. It is at this point when the treatment plan changes to focus on comfort care, or dying with dignity. Your doctor should review your options with you and include the option of hospice services at this time.

Hospice is a service that is comprised of designated staff that provides services specializing in end of life care. This involves preparing you, your family, and friends for the emotional and physical aspects of death. If you accept hospice care, you will be referred to the appropriate hospice program that will cater to your needs. This may include setting up hospice care in your own home, a hospice facility, or a hospital setting. The purpose of hospice care is to provide comfort, whether it is control of pain, medical equipment and other supplies, or spiritual or therapeutic counseling for the patient and family members. In addition, hospices coach caregivers on how to handle the patient's physical needs and offer respite care for caregivers.

When symptoms become too difficult, hospices provide short-term inpatient care; with the exception of pain medications, this typically means that you will no longer receive treatment for your cancer.

Hospice is a wonderful service that allows patients to focus on family and loved ones, instead of office visits and such, during their last days. The hospice staff also can help with the grieving process and provide counseling to your family members; spiritual needs can be addressed as well. Most importantly, hospice care is a way to reflect on your own life and your loved ones as you die peacefully.

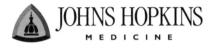

CHAPTER 10

Ovarian Cancer in Older Adults

By Gary R. Shapiro, MD

O varian cancer is primarily a disease of postmenopausal women and its frequency increases with
age. Contrary to what most people think, more
older women die from ovarian cancer than do younger
women. As we live longer, the number of women with ovarian cancer will increase dramatically. In the next 25 years,
the number of people who are 65 years of age and older will
double, and the largest increases in cancer incidence will
occur in those older than 80 years of age.

Older adults with cancer often have other chronic health
problems, and may be taking multiple medications that can
affect their cancer treatment plan. Prejudice, misunder-

standing, and limited access to clinical trials often prevent older patients from getting the timely cancer treatment that they need.

Older women may not have adequate evaluation of their symptoms, and when ovarian cancer is found, it is too often ignored or treated by suboptimal surgery and chemotherapy. As a result, older individuals often have more advanced stage cancer and worse outcomes than younger patients.

WHY IS THERE MORE CANCER IN OLDER PEOPLE?

The organs in our body are made up of cells. Cells divide and multiply as the body needs them. Cancer develops when cells in a part of the body grow out of control. The body has a number of ways of repairing damaged control mechanisms, but as we get older, these do not work as well. Although our healthier lifestyles have allowed us to avoid death from infection, heart attack, and stroke, we may now live long enough for a cancer to develop. People who live longer have increased exposure to cancer-causing agents (carcinogens) in the environment. Aging decreases the body's ability to protect us from these carcinogens and to repair cells that are damaged by these and other processes.

OVARIAN CANCER IS DIFFERENT IN OLDER WOMEN

The biology of ovarian cancer is different in older women than in younger women. As women age, their tumors are more aggressive and resistant to chemotherapy. In those with a family history or genetic predisposition (see Chapter 1), ovarian cancer typically occurs at a younger age. However, in women with BRCA mutations, the risk of ovarian, fallopian tube, or peritoneal cancer can occur at any age, including over 70.

DECISION MAKING: SEVEN PRACTICAL STEPS

1. GET A DIAGNOSIS

No matter how "typical" the signs and symptoms, first impressions are sometimes wrong.

Older women with unexplained abdominal symptoms are at high risk of a misdiagnosis, especially those with multiple medical problems and medications. Although ascites (fluid in the abdomen) is a classic sign of ovarian cancer, congestive heart failure and kidney disease can cause similar problems. Abdominal pain may be simple constipation, or some other type of cancer that requires completely different treatment than that used for cancer of the ovary. A diagnosis helps you and your family understand what to expect and how to prepare for the future, even if you cannot get curative treatment. Knowing the diagnosis also helps your doctor treat your symptoms better. Many people find "not knowing" very hard, and are relieved when they finally have an explanation for their symptoms. Sometimes a frail patient is obviously dying, and diagnostic studies can be an additional burden. In such cases, it may be quite reasonable to focus on symptom relief (palliation) without knowing the details of the diagnosis.

2. KNOW THE CANCER'S STAGE

The cancer's stage defines your prognosis and treatment options. No one can make informed decisions without it. Just as there may be times when the burdens of diagnostic studies may be too great, it may be appropriate to do without full staging in very frail, dying patients.

As it is in younger patients, stage is determined by the extent of the tumor, the presence or absence of cancer in the abdomen, or its spread (metastasis) to other organs. When doctors combine this information with information regarding your cancer's type and grade, and how much cancer remains after surgery, they can predict what impact, if any, your ovarian cancer is likely to have on your life expectancy and quality of life.

3. KNOW YOUR LIFE EXPECTANCY

Anticancer treatment should be considered if you are likely to live long enough to experience symptoms or premature death from ovarian cancer. If your life expectancy is so short that the cancer will not significantly affect it, there may be no reason to treat your cancer.

However, chronological age (how old you are) should not be the only thing that decides how your cancer should or should not be treated. Despite advanced age, women who are relatively well often have a life expectancy that is longer than their life expectancy with ovarian cancer. The average 70-year-old woman is likely to live another 16 years. A similar 85-year-old can expect to live an additional 6 years, and remain independent for most of that time. Even an unhealthy 75-year-old woman probably will live 5 more years; long enough to suffer symptoms and early death from metastatic ovarian cancer.

4. UNDERSTAND THE GOALS

Goals of Treatment

It is important to be clear whether the goal of treatment is cure (adjuvant therapy for ovarian cancer) or palliation (treatment for incurable recurrent or advanced metastatic ovarian cancer). If the goal is palliation, you need to understand if the treatment plan will extend your life, control your symptoms, or both. How likely is it to achieve these goals, and how long will you enjoy its benefits?

When the goal of treatment is palliation, chemotherapy should never be administered without defined endpoints and timelines. It should be clear to everyone what "counts" as success, how it will be determined (for example, a symptom controlled or a smaller mass on a CAT scan), and when. You and your family should understand what your options are at each step, and how likely each is to meet your goals. If this is not clear, ask your doctor to explain it in words that you understand.

Goals of the Patient

In addition to the traditional goals of tumor response, increased survival, and symptom control, older cancer patients often have goals related to quality of life. These may include physical and intellectual independence, spending quality time with your family, taking trips, staying out of the hospital, or even economic stability. At times, palliative care or hospice may meet these goals better than active anticancer treatment. In addition to the medical team, older patients often turn to family, friends, and clergy to help guide them.

5. DETERMINE IF YOU ARE FIT OR FRAIL

Deciding how to treat cancer in someone who is older requires a thorough understanding of her general health and social situation. Decisions about cancer treatment should never focus on age alone.

Age Is Not a Number

Your actual age (chronological age) has limited influence on how cancer will respond to therapy or its prognosis. Biological and other changes associated with aging are more reliable in estimating an individual's vigor, life expectancy, or the risk of treatment complications. These changes include malnutrition, loss of muscle mass and strength, depression, dementia, falls, social isolation, and the ability to accomplish daily activities such as dressing, bathing, eating, shopping, housekeeping, and managing one's finances or medication.

Chronic Illnesses

Older cancer patients are likely to have chronic illnesses (comorbidity) that affect their life expectancy; the more that you have, the greater the effect. This effect has very little impact on the behavior of the cancer itself, but studies do show that comorbidity has a major impact on treatment outcome and its side effects.

6. BALANCE BENEFITS AND HARMS

Fit older ovarian cancer patients respond to treatment similarly to their younger counterparts. However, a word of caution is in order. Until recently, few studies included older individuals, and it may not be appropriate to apply these findings to the diverse group of older cancer patients.

The side effects of cancer treatment are never less in the elderly. In addition to the standard side effects, there are significant age-related toxicities to consider. Though most of these are more a function of frailty than chronological age, even the fittest senior cannot avoid the physical effects of aging. In addition to the changes in fat and muscle that you see in the mirror, there are age-related changes in your kidney, liver, and digestive (gastrointestinal) function. These changes affect how your body absorbs and metabolizes anticancer drugs and other medicines. The average older woman takes many different medicines (to control, for example, high blood pressure, high cholesterol, osteoporosis, diabetes, arthritis, etc.). This "polypharmacy" can cause undesirable side effects as the many drugs interact with each other as well as with the anticancer medications.

7. GET INVOLVED

Healthcare providers and family members often underestimate the physical and mental abilities of older people and their willingness to face chronic and life-threatening conditions. Studies clearly show that older patients want detailed and easily understood information about potential treatments and alternatives. Patients and families may consider cancer untreatable in the aged, and not understand the possibilities offered by treatment.

While patients with dementia pose a unique challenge, they are frequently capable of participating in goal setting and simple discussions about treatment side effects and logistics. Caring family members and friends are often able to share the patient's life story so that healthcare workers can work with them to make decisions consistent with the patient's values and desires. This of course is no substitute for a well thought out and properly executed living will or healthcare proxy.

While it is hard to face the possibility of life-threatening events at any age, it is always better to be prepared and to "put your affairs in order." In addition to estate planning and wills, it is critical that you outline your wishes regarding medical care at the end of life, and make legal provisions for someone to make those decisions if you are unable to make them for yourself.

TREATING OVARIAN CANCER

YOU NEED A TEAM

Cancer care changes rapidly, and it is hard for the generalist to keep up to date, so referral to a specialist is essential. The needs of an older cancer patient often extend beyond the doctor's office and the traditional services provided by visiting nurses. These needs may include transportation, nutrition, emotional, financial, physical, or spiritual support. When an older woman with ovarian cancer is the primary caregiver for a frail or ill spouse, grandchildren, or other family members, special attention is necessary to provide for their needs as well. Older cancer patients cared for in geriatric oncology programs benefit from multidisciplinary teams of oncologists, geriatricians, psychiatrists, pharmacists, physiatrists, social workers, nurses, clergy, and dieticians, all working together as a team to identify and manage the stressors that can limit effective cancer treatment.

SURGERY

Cytoreductive debulking surgery is the standard of care for all women with ovarian cancer, regardless of age. Less aggressive surgery contributes to poorer outcomes in older women. Like other treatment options, ovarian cancer surgery in some older women may involve risks related to decreases in body organ (especially heart and lung) function, and it is essential that the surgeon and anesthetist work closely with your primary care physician (or a consultant) to fully assess and treat these problems before, during, and after the operation.

Surgery is as effective in elderly patients as in younger patients, but it does have a somewhat higher rate of complications in older individuals who have other medical problems (comorbidities). Neoadjuvant chemotherapy (see Chapter 3) is an option for some women who are not able to tolerate surgery, but it is not without its own risks. If an older person is too frail to undergo curative surgery, she is usually too frail to get chemotherapy. There are exceptions to this general rule, and it is essential that you weigh all of the risks and benefits with your multidisciplinary care team. Neoadjuvant chemotherapy is usually not a substitute for surgery, but it can serve to "buy time" for your doctors to get you ready for surgery by treating your other medical problems. It also can make for an "easier" operation, if your cancer responds to the chemotherapy.

RADIATION THERAPY

Radiation therapy is sometimes used after an isolated recurrence is surgically removed, but it has no role in first-line therapy for women with ovarian cancer. It provides excellent symptom relief (palliation) in metastatic and other incurable situations. It is particularly effective in treating pain caused by ovarian cancer metastases to the bone. A short course of radiation therapy often allows patients with advanced cancer to lower (or even eliminate) their dose of narcotic pain relievers. Although these medicines do an excellent job of controlling pain, they often cause confusion, falls, and constipation in older patients. Thus, even hospice patients suffering from localized metastatic bone pain should consider the option of palliative radiation therapy.

Though studies in older women have found no significant increase in the side effects from radiation therapy, the fatigue that often accompanies radiation therapy can be quite profound in the elderly, even in those who are fit. Often the logistical details (like daily travel to the hospital for a six-week course of treatment) are the hardest for older people. It is important that you discuss these potential problems with your family and social worker prior to starting radiation therapy. Women who have cardiac pacemakers may need to have them moved to a location outside of the radiation therapy fields to avoid pacemaker malfunctions during treatment.

CHEMOTHERAPY

Non-frail older cancer patients respond to chemotherapy similarly to their younger counterparts. Reducing the dose of chemotherapy based purely on chronological age may seriously affect the effectiveness of treatment. Managing chemotherapy-associated toxicity with appropriate supportive care is crucial in the elderly population to give them the best chance of cure and survival, or to provide the best palliation.

Though the side effects of cancer treatment are never less burdensome in the elderly, they can be managed by oncologists, especially geriatric oncologists, who work in teams with others who specialize in the care of the elderly. With appropriate care, healthy older patients do just as well with chemotherapy as younger patients. Advances in supportive care (antinausea medicines and blood cell growth factors) have significantly decreased the side effects of chemotherapy, and improved safety and the quality of life of individuals with ovarian cancer. Nonetheless, there is risk, especially if the patient is frail. The presence of severe comorbidities, age-related frailty, or underlying severe psychosocial problems may be obstacles for highly intensive treatment plans. Such patients may benefit from less complicated or potentially less toxic treatment plans.

With regard to choice of chemotherapy, healthy older patients can receive the same adjuvant regimens as their younger counterparts. If you can tolerate cytoreductive surgery, you can usually tolerate combination platinum-taxane chemotherapy (see Chapter 3). These standard adjuvant treatment programs are particularly important when the goal of treatment is cure.

Studies have shown that doctors often under-treat older women with potentially curable ovarian cancers. Though the desire to minimize side effects is understandable, these doctors are not doing you any favors. Adjuvant chemotherapy is significantly less effective when it is given in lower than standard doses or when treatment is delayed. Because the goal of adjuvant chemotherapy is cure, every effort should be taken to avoid delay and dose reductions.

Older women whose ovarian cancers have progressed despite first-line therapy have the same benefit from additional chemotherapy as their younger counterparts. They should not be excluded from receiving chemotherapy for recurrent ovarian cancer. When chemotherapy is being used to control (palliate) recurrent or metastatic ovarian cancer, preference should be given to chemotherapeutic drugs with safer profiles, single-agent regimens, low-dose weekly schedules, or even dose reductions. Many oncologists favor Doxil or weekly Hycamtin, but there are many other active regimens like Paraplatin, Taxotere, Taxol, Gemzar, VePesid (oral etoposide), or Toposar (oral etoposide).

The benefits of cisplatin-based intraperitoneal chemotherapy (see Chapter 3) are across all age groups. Nevertheless, a word of caution is in order when considering older women for this form of adjuvant treatment. One of the major side effects of Platinol AQ is kidney damage. Because kidney function decreases with age, severe side effects are more common in older patients than those who are younger. As long as kidney function is carefully monitored, it seems reasonable to consider this promising treatment in older women who are not frail.

HORMONAL THERAPY

Although only a very small number of women have ovarian cancer that respond to hormonal therapy, these agents may be worth a try in woman with advanced ovarian cancer who are too frail to get chemotherapy. To determine if you have this type of ovarian cancer, a pathologist will analyze your cancer tissue specimen or biopsy to see if it contains hormone (estrogen or progesterone) receptors. If it does, you and your doctor may decide to try an antiestrogen pill like Soltamox or Arimidex (one of a class of drugs called aromatase inhibitors). Although you might experience hot flashes, sweating or muscle cramps when you start these medicines, most women usually tolerate them quite well. Hormonal therapy may be worth a try for frail women with advanced, recurrent, hormone receptor positive ovarian cancer. However, it should never be used for women who can tolerate palliative chemotherapy or those with potentially curable ovarian cancer.

COMMON TREATMENT COMPLICATIONS IN THE ELDERLY

Anemia (low red blood cell count) is common in the elderly, especially the frail elderly. It decreases the effectiveness of chemotherapy, and often causes fatigue, falls, cognitive decline (for example, dementia, disorientation or confusion) and heart problems. Therefore, it is essential that anemia be recognized and corrected with red blood cell transfusions or the appropriate use of erythropoiesis-stimulating agents like Procrit and Epogen or Aranesp.

Myelosuppression (low white blood cell count) is also common in older patients getting chemotherapy or radiation therapy. Older patients with myelosuppression develop life-threatening infections more often than younger patients, and they may need to be treated in the hospital for many days. The liberal use of granulopoietic growth factors (G-CSF, Neupogen, Neulasta) decreases the risk of infection, and makes it possible for older women to receive full doses of potentially curable adjuvant chemotherapy.

Mucositis (mouth sores) and diarrhea can cause severe dehydration in older patients who often are already dehydrated due to inadequate fluid intake and diuretics ("water pills" for high blood pressure or heart failure). Careful monitoring and the liberal use of antidiarrheal agents (Imodium) and oral and intravenous fluids are essential components of the management of older cancer patients. Chemotherapy induced nausea and vomiting can contribute to dehydration, and it is essential that elderly patients receive enough medicine (antiemetics) to control this loss of fluids. Nausea and vomiting is especially problematic for patients getting Platinol AQ.

Other gastrointestinal side effects, including pain and obstruction, can be caused by surgery or chemotherapy. The resulting constipation can be particularly difficult to manage in elderly patients who are prone to this problem. The dehydration and poor appetite that often accompany chemotherapy can make constipation worse. Maintaining adequate nutrition and fluid intake, and careful use of stool softeners and laxatives are essential.

Kidney function declines as we age. Some of the medicines that older patients take to treat both their cancer (for example, Platinol AQ, Paraplatin, Reclast [zoledronic acid], NSAIDs) and noncancer related problems might make this worse. The dehydration that often accompanies cancer and its treatment can put additional stress on the kidneys. Fortunately, it is often possible to minimize these effects by carefully selecting and dosing appropriate drugs, managing "polypharmacy," and preventing dehydration.

Neurotoxicity and cognitive effects (chemo-brain) can be profoundly debilitating in patients who are already cognitively impaired (demented, disoriented, confused, etc.). Elderly patients with a history of falling, hearing loss, or peripheral neuropathy (for example, nerve damage from diabetes) have decreased energy and are highly vulnerable to neurotoxic chemotherapy like the taxanes or platinum compounds. Many of the medicines used to control nausea (antiemetics) or decrease the side effects of certain chemotherapeutic agents are also potential neurotoxins. These include Decadron (dexamethasone) for psychosis and agitation, Zantac (ranitidine) for agitation, Benadryl, and some of the antiemetics (sedation).

Fatigue is a near universal complaint of older cancer patients. It is particularly a problem for those who are socially isolated or depend upon others to help them with activities of daily living. It is not necessarily related to depression, but can be. Depression is quite common in the elderly. In contrast to younger patients who often respond to a cancer diagnosis with anxiety, depression is the more common disorder in older cancer patients. With proper support and medical attention, many of these patients can safely receive anticancer treatment.

Heart problems increase with age, and it is no surprise that older cancers patients have an increased risk of cardiac complications from intensive surgery, radiation, and chemotherapy. Patients treated with Platinol AQ chemotherapy require large amounts of intravenous fluid hydration. This can cause congestive heart failure in patients with heart problems, so they need careful monitoring. One should also keep in mind the cardiovascular complications that hormonal therapies such as Soltamox can cause, especially blood clots (thrombosis).

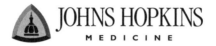

CHAPTER 11

TRUSTED RESOURCES— FINDING ADDITIONAL INFORMATION ABOUT OVARIAN CANCER AND ITS TREATMENT

Johns Hopkins Ovarian Cancer Center of Excellence
   http://www.ovariancancercenter.org
   (410) 955-8240

The goal of the Johns Hopkins Ovarian Cancer Center of Excellence is to improve the care of women with ovarian cancer. They provide comprehensive ovarian cancer services including prevention, screening, diagnosis, treatment, and access to the latest and most promising therapies. They promote research that develops innovative and improved methods for diagnosing and treating this disease. The Web site also contains information on research, clinical trials, support services and contact information.

National Cancer Institute

http://www.cancer.gov/cancertopics/types/ovarian

(800) 4-CANCER

This Web site provides an overview on ovarian cancer from the definition to treatment options. There is information on clinical trials that are available as well as up-to-date literature on ovarian cancer. You can also find information on genetics, risk-reducing options, and they provide an online book entitled, *What You Need to Know About Ovarian Cancer*. You can request free information by calling the toll-free number.

American Cancer Society

http://www.cancer.org/docroot/lrn/lrn_0.asp

(800) ACS-2345

This link provides educational information on ovarian cancer (glossary of terms, treatment, and statistics), provides available sources of information, and allows you to read other people's experiences as well as share your own.

National Ovarian Cancer Coalition (NOCC)

http://www.ovarian.org

E-mail: NOCC@ovarian.com

(888) OVARIAN

This organization's mission is to raise awareness and promote education to increase the survival rate and quality of life for women with ovarian cancer. They provide basic information on ovarian cancer as well as updates in the medical literature. There are available resources (particularly on local/state chapters) listed on the Web site, and they offer many options for you to become involved in the fight against ovarian cancer.

National Coalition for Cancer Survivorship

http://www.canceradvocacy.org

(877) 622-7937

The National Coalition for Cancer Survivorship is the oldest survivor-led cancer advocacy organization in the country. They stand for quality cancer care and empowering cancer survivors. They focus on changes at the federal level for how the nation researches, regulates, finances, and delivers quality cancer care. They also place a large focus on patient education and provide an educational audio program entitled the Cancer Survival Toolbox®.

Ovarian Cancer National Alliance

http://www.ovariancancer.org

(866) 399-6262 / 202-331-1332

This organization's mission is to conquer ovarian cancer by uniting individuals and organizations into a national movement. In addition to information on ovarian cancer, they provide resources and a national calendar of events that support ovarian cancer research.

Johns Hopkins Pathology

http://www.ovariancancer.jhmi.edu/

This Johns Hopkins Web site provides information on ovarian cancer as well as summaries of major research in the field. They also provide insights into patient perspectives and information on upcoming events and occasionally a photo gallery. They also have information on obtaining an appointment, clinical trials, and hospital information.

American Society of Clinical Oncology (ASCO)
http://www.oncology.com
(703) 299-0150

This organization provides an overview of all cancers where you can specifically view ovarian cancer as well as the top advances in cancer research. There is also information on learning about cancer, statistics, upcoming events, and links to major cancer journals. They also provide podcasts of recent events in the field of cancer care.

Cancer Care, Inc.
http://www.cancercare.org
(800) 813-HOPE

This is a national not-for-profit organization that provides free, professional support services for anyone affected by cancer (regardless of type). In addition to information for the patient, they also provide information for family and loved ones including education, counseling, financial information and assistance for non-medical expenses, and referrals for additional services.

Gilda Radner Familial Ovarian Cancer Registry
http://www.ovariancancer.com
(800) OVARIAN

This is an international registry of families affected by ovarian cancer (two or more relatives). They also offer a hotline, newsletter, and informational pamphlets. Their goal is to pursue research, particularly in familial ovarian cancer cases. They support research in this area as well as psycho-social counseling for families and individuals.

Gilda's Club

http://www.gildasclub.org

(800) GILDA4U

Gilda's Club has the mission of providing free support for anyone living with cancer as well as their family and friends. They complement medical care by providing networking and support groups, educational and social activities, and workshops.

Look Good . . . Feel Better

http://www.lookgoodfeelbetter.org

(800) 395-LOOK

This Web site provides information on ways to find resources and provides tips on maintaining a healthy and beautiful outward appearance for women with cancer. This includes hair products (wigs, accessories) to make-up tips, as well as other information.

Society of Gynecologic Oncologists (SGO)

http://www.sgo.org

(800) 444-4441

This society's mission is to promote and ensure the highest quality of comprehensive clinical care, education, and research in gynecologic cancers with the goal of eradicating these diseases. This Web site provides information on up-to-date research and links to find a gynecologic oncologist near you.

Ovarian Cancer Research Fund, Inc. (OCRF)
http://www.ocrf.org
(800) 873-9569

The mission of the OCRF is to fund research in efforts to find a method of early detection and ultimately a cure for ovarian cancer. This Web site provides information on national events, insights into ongoing research, and opportunities to donate to this program.

SHARE: Self-help for women with breast or ovarian cancer
http://www.sharecancersupport.org
(212) 719-0364
(866) 891-2392

This is an organization (English and Spanish speaking) that provides support to ovarian and breast cancer survivors through hotlines, support groups, educational programs, and activities. They advocate for women's health issues on a national forum to support research for these two conditions.

Patient Advocate Foundation
http://www.patientadvocate.org
E-mail: patient@pinn.net
(800) 532-5274 / (757) 873-6668

This is a national not-for-profit organization that helps patients obtain access to care, insurance assistance, maintenance of employment, and financial stability.

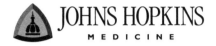

INFORMATION ABOUT JOHNS HOPKINS

The Johns Hopkins Ovarian Cancer Center of Excellence
Appointment Line: (410) 502-4245
http://www.ovariancancercenter.org

The goal of the Johns Hopkins Ovarian Cancer Center of Excellence is to reduce the mortality and morbidity of ovarian cancer. We provide comprehensive ovarian cancer services including prevention, screening, diagnosis, treatment, and access to the latest and most promising therapies. Patients have access to cutting edge early detection techniques through the Breast and Ovarian Surveillance Service (BOSS Clinic). Our gynecologic oncologists have extensive experience in the full range of surgical treatments for ovarian cancer, including the use of minimally invasive approaches as well as more extensive cytoreductive (debulking) operations for patients with more advanced or recurrent disease. Our services are accessible, high quality, and treat the entire patient with a holistic approach. The Ovarian Cancer Center promotes research that develops innovative and improved methods for diagnosing and treating this disease. Our website address is **http://www.ovariancancercenter.org** and contains information on ovarian cancer risk factors, diagnosis, and treatment of newly diagnosed and recurrent disease. The site also contains information on genetic risk assessment and testing, available clinical trials, useful supportive services, and links to NCCN Practice Guidelines and upcoming conferences. We also have mechanisms on the website for obtaining second opinions and requesting physician-to-physician consultations.

About Johns Hopkins Medicine

Johns Hopkins Medicine unites physicians and scientists of The Johns Hopkins University School of Medicine with the organizations, health professionals, and facilities of the Johns Hopkins Health System. Its mission is to improve the health of the community and the world by setting the standard of excellence in medical education, research, and clinical care. Diverse and inclusive, Johns Hopkins Medicine has provided international leadership in the education of physicians and medical scientists in biomedical research and in the application of medical knowledge to sustain health since The Johns Hopkins Hospital opened in 1889.

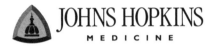

FURTHER READING

100 Questions and Answers About Ovarian Cancer, Second Edition, Don S. Dizon & Nadeem R. Abu-Rustum, Jones and Bartlett Publishers, 2007.

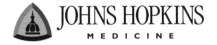

GLOSSARY

Acute-onset nausea and vomiting: A queasy or upset stomach and then emptying of stomach matter through the mouth that usually occurs immediately or in a short time frame after receiving chemotherapy.

Adjuvant therapy: Treatment given after the primary surgery to increase the chances of a cure, and treatment to prevent remission.

Advance directives: Legal documents that detail the decisions of a patient in the event of a terminal event (i.e., what they do and do not want to have done during their last weeks or months) in case they become unable to communicate effectively.

Alopecia: Loss of hair.

Alternative therapy: Complementary medicine therapies used with, or instead of, standard medical therapies; these include herbal remedies, acupuncture, etc.

Anemia: Decrease in the number of red blood cells (can result in fatigue).

Antiemetics: Antinausea medications.

Antihormones: A class of drugs that block hormones before they can bind to the receptors in a tumor.

Ascites: Abnormal buildup of fluid in the abdomen.

Biopsy: A minor procedure in which cells are collected for microscopic examination by a pathologist.

Cancer: The presence of malignant cells.

Carcinomas: Cancers that form in the surface cells of different tissues.

Chemotherapy (cytotoxic therapy): The use of chemical agents (drugs) to systematically treat cancer.

Clinical trial: A study of a drug or treatment with a large group of people testing the treatment.

Cytoreductive surgery: A type of surgery performed to remove as much of the cancerous tissue as possible. There are two types, optimal and suboptimal. Upon completion of optimal cytoreduction, there are no cancerous tissue deposits measuring larger than 1 cm. At the completion of suboptimal cytoreduction, there are cancerous tissue deposits greater than 1 cm.

Cytotoxic: The ability to kill fast growing cells, both cancerous and noncancerous, by preventing them from dividing.

Debulking: Another term for cytoreductive surgery.

Delayed-onset vomiting: Develops more than 24 hours after chemotherapy is given.

Durable power of attorney: Allows a specific family member to legally make all your decisions, personal and financial, for you in case you become incapacitated.

Endocrine therapy: See *hormonal therapy*.

Epithelial: Cells on the surface of a tissue.

Estrogen: One of the major female hormones secreted by the ovary.

Fertility preservation: Leaving the uterus and at least part of one ovary to allow for future child-bearing.

Genetic predisposition: An increased risk of having a genetic mutation inherited from a parent that can result in a higher risk for developing a medical condition.

Healthcare proxy: A legal document that permits a designated person to make decisions regarding your medical treatment when you are unable to do so.

Histologic grade (or tumor grade): A microscopic examination of tumor cells that describes how slow or fast the cancer cells are growing.

Hormonal therapy: Treatment that blocks the effects of hormones upon cancers that depend on hormones to grow (also referred to as endocrine therapy).

Hormone replacement therapy: Administration of artificial estrogen and progesterone to alleviate the symptoms of menopause and to prevent health problems experienced by postmenopausal women, particularly osteoporosis.

Incidence: The number of times a disease occurs within a population of people.

Informed consent: A process by which patients undergoing surgery or participating in a clinical study are provided with all available information prior to agreeing to receive that treatment.

Intraperitoneal (IP) catheter: A device that is placed underneath the skin, on the lower portion of the ribcage, and connected to a tube that goes into the abdominal cavity. It is used to deliver chemotherapy directly into the abdomen.

Invasive cancer: A type of aggressive cancer that breaks through normal tissue barriers and invades surrounding areas.

Living will: A legal document that outlines what care you want in the event you become unable to communicate due to coma or heavy sedation.

Lymph nodes: Tissues in the lymphatic system that filter lymph fluid and help the immune system fight disease.

Lymphatic system: A collection of vessels with the principal functions of transporting digested fat from the intestine to the blood stream, removing and destroying toxins from tissues, and resisting the spread of disease throughout the body.

Malignant: A type of cancer that grows rapidly and out of control.

Menopause: End of menstrual periods.

Metastasis, metastasize: The spread of cancer to other organ sites.

Mortality: The statistical calculation of death rates due to a specific disease within a population.

Mutation: A gene with an alteration.

Narcotics: A class of pain medications requiring a prescription (e.g., morphine, codeine).

Neoadjuvant therapy: Therapy that is started before the primary treatment.

Neuropathy: A disorder of the peripheral nerves that may cause intermittent numbness, tingling, weakness, and pain in the hands and feet.

Neutropenia: A condition of an abnormally low number of a particular type of white blood cell, called a neutrophil, that may result in an increased risk of infection.

Nonsteroidal anti-inflammatory drugs (NSAIDs): A class of pain medications (e.g., ibuprofen).

Omentum: A fold of fatty tissue that surrounds the stomach/colon and other organs in the abdomen.

Oncologist: A degreed, board-eligible/certified physician specializing in the identification and treatment of cancer (tumors).

Optimal cytoreduction: See *cytoreductive surgery.*

Palliative care: Comfort care provided to relieve the symptoms of cancer and to keep the best quality of life for as long as possible without seeking to cure the disease.

Paracentesis: Removing fluid (ascites) from the abdomen using a needle to obtain a diagnosis or provide relief.

Pathologist: A degreed, board-eligible/certified physician specialist trained to distinguish normal from abnormal cells.

Peritoneal washings: Sterile fluid introduced and removed from the abdomen and pelvis at the time of surgery to look for microscopic spread of cancer cells within this area.

Peritoneum: The lining of the abdominal cavity and surrounds the organs within the abdomen.

Platelets: Components of blood that assist in clotting.

Pleural effusion: Fluid collection around lungs.

Port: A catheter placed in a vein to allow for blood draws as well as the administration of medications (may also be placed in the peritoneal cavity for medication administration only).

Primary care doctor: A physician who performs routine check-ups.

Primary prevention: Any treatment method or lifestyle change that directly prevents cancer cells from forming, growing, or multiplying.

Progesterone: A major female hormone produced by the ovary.

Prognosis: An estimation of the likely outcome of an illness based upon the patient's current status and the available treatments.

Protocol: The research plan for how the drug is given and to whom it is given.

Recurrent cancer: When the disease has returned despite the initial treatment.

Red blood cells: Cells in the blood with the primary function of carrying oxygen to tissues.

Refractory cancer: Cancer that has not responded to treatment.

Risk factors: Any factors that contribute to an increased possibility of getting cancer.

Stage: A numerical determination of how far the cancer has progressed.

Suboptimal cytoreduction: See *cytoreductive surgery.*

Targeted therapy: Treatment that targets specific molecules involved in carcinogenesis or tumor growth.

Tumor: Abnormal mass or lump of tissue.

Ultrasonography: An imaging technique that uses sound waves to determine whether a mass is solid or fluid-filled, or a combination of the two.

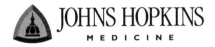

INDEX